W0113256

Towards a Transtheoret[ical] Definition of Countertra[nsference]

This book explores the analyst's countertransfe[rence] settings from a number of theoretical perspect[ives] transtheoretical definition of countertransference.

Stemming from an examination of the definiti[on] itself, the author utilizes a philosophical hermene[utic] pathological countertransference develops, how an[alysts] from the patient's experience, and what analysts s[hould] countertransference response from interfering wit[h] unique hermeneutic methodology, philosophical writings are explored as a way of gaining a deeper me[aning] of countertransference. By re-interpreting these new light, the book develops a transtheoretical defi[nition of] countertransference. As such, the author offers a tim[ely] meaning and understanding of countertransference as it [has] century, going from being considered an obstacle to trea[tment] analyst's unconscious conflicts to being understood as a [way] and understanding the patient's unconscious material. It pathway through various depth psychological, therap[eutic] approaches to countertransference, foregrounding t[he] therapeutic value of the concept and seeking a new transt[heoretical]

This volume will appeal to scholars and researchers mental health.

Dr. Rudy Roman is a clinical assistant professor of behavioral sciences with Keck School of Medicine of the Un[iversity of Southern] California, USA, and an adjunct assistant professor with the also at the University of Southern California, USA. He has a Long Beach, California, USA, and has been providing men[tal health services] for over 14 years.

Explor[ing...]

Towards a Transtheoretical Definition of Countertransference

Re-visioning the Clinician's Intersubjective Experience

Rudy Roman

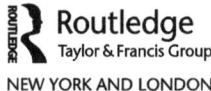

NEW YORK AND LONDON

First published 2023
by Routledge
605 Third Avenue, New York, NY 10158

and by Routledge
4 Park Square, Milton Park, Abingdon, Oxon, OX14 4RN

Routledge is an imprint of the Taylor & Francis Group, an informa business

Library of Congress Cataloging-in-Publication Data
Names: Roman, Rudy, author.
Title: Towards a transtheoretical definition of countertransference : re-visioning
   the clinician's intersubjective experience / Rudy Roman.
Description: First edition. | New York, NY : Routledge, 2023. |
   Series: Explorations in mental health | Includes bibliographical
   references and index.
Identifiers: LCCN 2022036589 (print) | LCCN 2022036590 (ebook) |
   ISBN 9781032335568 (hbk) | ISBN 9781032335582 (pbk) |
   ISBN 9781003320180 (ebk)
Subjects: LCSH: Countertransference (Psychology)
Classification: LCC RC489.C68 R64 2023 (print) | LCC RC489.C68 (ebook) |
   DDC 616.89/14—dc23/eng/20220912
LC record available at https://lccn.loc.gov/2022036589
LC ebook record available at https://lccn.loc.gov/2022036590

ISBN: 978-1-032-33556-8 (hbk)
ISBN: 978-1-032-33558-2 (pbk)
ISBN: 978-1-003-32018-0 (ebk)

DOI: 10.4324/9781003320180

Typeset in Times New Roman
by Apex CoVantage, LLC

Para mis padres, Emilio y Guadalupe Roman

and
To my pride and joy, my son, James Daniel Roman

Contents

Acknowledgments

I would like to express my sincerest gratitude to those who played a role in making this book possible. To Dr. Marybeth Carter, Dr. Christine Lewis, and Dr. Edward Rounds for their nurturance and supportive approach during the writing process. I will always be grateful for your knowledge, commitment, and dedication throughout the process. To my son James Daniel Roman for being my daily motivator throughout the process. I do not have words to express my love for you. You are my everything, and I love you with all my heart! To my father Emilio Roman and my sister Ruth Roman for always pushing me to strive for greatness. Both of you have served as an inspiration not only through your love but also by serving as examples of greatness yourselves. Thank you for always believing in me. I love you both very much. To my mother Guadalupe Roman and my sister Virginia "Gina" Hassouneh for loving me unconditionally and providing me with the opportunity to experience the true meaning of love. Both of you are examples of the ideal mother, and I will always love you as you have loved me. To my brother-in-law Amer Hassouneh for being such a wonderful, supportive, and loving man. You have served as an example of what it takes to be a model husband, father, and man, and I am grateful to have you in my life. To Tania Valtierra for pushing me and helping me get across the finish line. I am eternally grateful for your support and encouraging ways when I needed it the most. You believed in me and I will always be grateful for that. To my mentor Dr. Jack Wasserman for his guidance through one of the most difficult phases of my life. You have been an inspirational presence in my life, and I will always be grateful for that. To Marsha Welch and Dr. Henry Drummond for always pushing me to become the best version of myself. To Ronald "Chris" Bagley for always believing in me and what I am capable of being, not only from a professional and academic standpoint but as a person as well. To Adrian Romero, whom I have known for the past 25 years. Thank you for always encouraging me and for being a rock I could lean on. To my classmate Bryce McDavitt. Although we had our differences while attending Pacifica Graduate Institute, you made yourself available in sharing your knowledge and helping me understand things I may have found confusing during the writing process. Thank you, my friend. And finally, to my higher power for guiding me through the process and giving me the strength to persevere and never quit.

Introduction

The concept of countertransference has been a controversial topic since its introduction by Sigmund Freud in the early 1900s. The meaning and understanding of countertransference have evolved over time; however, a standard definition still does not exist. The Freudian drive model encouraged the avoidance of the analyst's emotional response as it reflected the analyst's unmet drive-related conflicts (Freud, 1910/1953). Later, the examination of the analyst's subjective experience in regard to their emotional response represented a shared experience with the patient and reflected the patient's unconscious material (Natterson, 1991). Although psychodynamic approaches tend to focus more on this phenomenon, having a subjective response to patient material is universal and inevitable, as well as being a part of psychotherapy regardless of theoretical orientation. Therefore, it is valuable to be knowledgeable about how the spectrum of theoretical orientations works with the phenomenon.

When examining the range of countertransference perspectives, the initial views of the phenomenon centered on the Freudian drive model. Freud's understanding of countertransference developed from his work with patients and what appeared to be the patient's unconscious redirection of feelings or affect toward the analyst. Freud explained that this "transferring" of feelings was related to an early life experience by the patient, with the affect transferred belonging to another person within the patient's experience. Freud called this phenomenon *transference* and considered it a portal into the patient's unconscious as it provided a greater understanding of the patient's unconscious phantasies and innate drives (Freud, 1912/1953). Since countertransference was seen as simply transference on behalf of the analyst, countertransference was considered an interference with treatment as a result of the analyst's own infantile drive-related conflicts triggered by the patient (Greenberg & Mitchell, 1983). As a result, Freud stressed that analysts need to overcome and vigilantly resist their countertransference response, even when the urge to indulge in it presented itself by way of their narcissistic need. Freud deemed countertransference a deviation from the central tenet of the "objective neutrality" of the analyst (Freud, 1915/1958). Although Freud eventually came to the conclusion that "everyone possesses in his own unconscious an instrument with which he can interpret the utterances of the unconscious in other people," countertransference

DOI: 10.4324/9781003320180-1

and the idea of the analyst's unconscious serving as a therapeutic tool remained a concept commonly overlooked and avoided by Freud (Favero & Ross, 2002, p. 221). Many argued that Freud's avoidance was related to his negative views on countertransference and his concern about others becoming aware of his own infantile drive-related conflicts (Gelso & Hayes, 2007).

Stern (1924) continued with the Freudian drive model of countertransference and considered it "the transference that the analyst makes to the patient" brought on by the repressed libidinal urges stemming from the analyst's childhood (p. 167). In other words, the origins of countertransference were the same as transference: the analyst's repressed libidinal needs or unresolved neurotic difficulties. Ferenczi and Rank (1923) added an additional layer to the fold and considered the analyst's narcissist response as a form of countertransference. As a result, two distinct concepts began to emerge: countertransference was either the analyst's response to the patient's transference or a response triggered by the analyst's own unresolved issues (Orr, 1954).

By 1927, ideas concerning countertransference were moving away from the classic drive theory; however, this was not the general consensus of the time (Orr, 1954). Like those before him, Glover (1924) compared countertransference to transference: just as positive and negative transferences occur, the same could be said about countertransference (Orr, 1954). Reich (1947), however, returned to the classic drive model and considered countertransference to be a result of the unresolved issues of the analyst. Although many theorists such as Horney and the Balints followed, the first real challenge to the classic drive theory of countertransference occurred almost two decades later.

During the 1950s, there was a paradigm shift resulting in a wider range of opinions on countertransference. Many theorists such as Winnicott, Heimann, Little, and Racker (all later discussed in greater detail) challenged classic drive theory, considering countertransference as a tool accessible for the analyst to become more knowledgeable of the patient's unconscious, allowing for a greater understanding of the patient's experiences and unconscious processes (Zachrisson, 2009). Although Freud, like many of his predecessors, held a strong belief that countertransference was a permanent problem because it could pull analysts away from their ability to remain objective, the latter view was embraced and accepted, and considered countertransference to be a useful tool in better understanding the patient (Karamanolaki, 2008). The perspectives on countertransference were no longer focusing strictly on the classic drive model but instead were examining the analyst's experience of the patient as a way of gaining a deeper understanding of the patient's internal world. Natterson (1991) added, "the subjective experience of both patient and therapist are indispensable ingredients of the therapeutic phenomenon" (p. 21). For Natterson, the inter-subjective experience of the analyst served as a way of connecting the analyst with the experience of the patient. When such a connection is made, there is a deeper understanding on behalf of the analyst of the patient's experience, hence providing greater "relatability" due to the shared experience between the patient and the analyst (Natterson, 1991). Although advancements have been made to form new ways to understand countertransference, countertransference remains linked with outdated perspectives that do not take into account the emotional involvement or the subjective experience of the analyst, both of which are an intricate part of the analytic process (Gelso & Hayes, 2007).

The Researcher's Predisposition to the Topic

My interest in countertransference began during my master's-level practicum at Glendale Memorial Hospital. While learning about countertransference, most readings and lectures I was exposed to describe countertransference as negative in nature, a phenomenon that would hinder the therapeutic process, and require the analyst to refer the patient. One of the most common definitions of countertransference used within my master's studies was that of Murdock. Murdock (2004) writes:

> Countertransference is what happens when the therapist has not had a proper training analysis. Conflicts from the counselor's past are projected into the analytic situation, and the therapist loses her objectivity. The client becomes "special" to the counselor (a positive countertransference), or the therapist begins to want to argue or gets angry with the client. The counselor may find herself looking forward to or dreading seeing a particular client. The only way to resolve countertransference is for the analyst to seek the aid of her training analyst or a professional consultant.
>
> (pp. 53–54)

According to Murdock (2004), countertransference was a hindrance to treatment resulting in the analyst's unresolved issues becoming the focal point of treatment. In other words, therapy was no longer about the patient but about the analyst. My first job as a therapist was in a context that paralleled Murdock's view of countertransference. This perspective was also the position of the county program for which I worked: countertransference is negative and to be avoided. However, while attending my doctoral program, I began reading about a completely different approach to countertransference, which stimulated my intellectual curiosity. In my studies of depth psychology, countertransference was seen as possibly beneficial to the therapeutic relationship. I was fascinated by this approach to countertransference and the variety of perspectives offered depending on the theoretical orientation. However, although there were many different descriptions of the phenomenon, there was no clear-cut answer or middle ground: Countertransference was to be embraced or eliminated. At the same time, I was experiencing difficulties related to countertransference in working with an adult patient.

Autobiographical Origins of the Researcher's Interest in the Topic

Although I had a rudimentary understanding of the concept of countertransference and how to use it to assist with the transference/countertransference dynamic within sessions, I was conflicted when working with an adult female patient on my caseload because I was unable to explain or understand my immense dislike and uneasiness while in session with her.

One day, my morning was as uneventful as any other. Knowing I had my usual Tuesday morning appointment with my patient of almost 1 year, I did my usual routine of answering emails, returning phone calls, and reviewing the note from our previous session before her arrival. After greeting her in the lobby and walking her to my office, the session began the way it usually did with my talking with her about her difficulty in limiting her alcohol consumption and changing her unsafe sexual practices. However, during the session I felt an intense feeling of anxiety and a sense of unwanted energy coming toward me from her, and spoke of it. She responded by saying, "I have an attraction to teenage boys" with the look of a little girl fantasizing about her prince charming. Immediately upon hearing her words, I froze and began to feel fear. I looked at her and felt disgust and hatred. Not knowing if this reaction was brought on by her comment or a psychic energy coming into the room, I chose to refrain from commenting on my reaction, especially given that I was more concerned about assessing for potential child abuse. Fortunately, my assessment did not identify any current or potential victims. With each subsequent session, my feelings and reactions intensified to the point that I no longer wanted to work with the patient. I knew I was struggling with countertransference; however, I could not understand why I became overwhelmed by these feelings or what was causing them. Unsure of what to think or do, I turned to my clinical supervisor for guidance and support.

While discussing the case with my clinical supervisor, I frequently mentioned my hatred toward this client, a hatred that suddenly and unexplainably came on. Although we looked at the case from different angles in hopes of uncovering and resolving my difficulties, I could not link or understand my difficulties with and immense feelings toward this patient until my clinical supervisor asked me an unexpected question: "Rudy, have you ever been molested?" My initial response to his question was one of anger and disbelief. I said, "Of course not!" He again asked, "Are you sure?" My anger intensified when I was asked the same question, and I said, "Of course not! How would I not remember being molested?" At that point, I remembered a childhood memory that had been repressed for over 20 years: I remembered Steve, the man who befriended me as a child and attempted to molest me.

As a seventh-grade boy, I was befriended by my friend's neighbor Steve. Steve was a competitive weightlifter, and I gravitated toward him, especially since I was a big sports fan who looked up to the athletes of the time. Like most kids my age, I wanted to "be like Mike" and fantasized about someday leading my beloved Phoenix Suns to their first NBA championship. I had dreams of becoming a professional athlete. Steve frequently joined the neighborhood kids for a game of football, displaying his superior strength for all of us to see. Steve also took the time to give my friend and me a ride to the Boys and Girls Club for our basketball practices while also sliding us a few dollars so we could buy snacks after practice. Steve was not just my friend's neighbor but *my* friend, a parental figure, and someone I trusted.

One day while on my way to the Boys and Girls Club, I stopped by my friend's house to see if he wanted to come along, but to my surprise, he wasn't home. Thinking he might be at Steve's house, I chose to go across the street. Once Steve realized it was me, he invited me in. This was the first time I had ever been in his house. As I looked around, I was surrounded by pictures and trophies from his competitions. Seeing the look of amazement on my face, Steve asked me if I was interested in "getting like that." Steve was referring to his physique in a picture I was looking at of him at a weightlifting competition. After I expressed my desire to get stronger in hopes of getting closer to my dream of becoming a professional athlete, he said, "Why don't you take off your shirt?" At the time I was confused by his request because I knew he was wrong to ask such a thing of me. My parents always warned me against predators, but in my eyes, Steve wasn't a predator, he was my friend. I stood there, confused, and not knowing what to do. Steve looked at me, smiled and said, "Go ahead, take off your shirt." Not knowing what to do, I complied and took off my shirt. As I stood there – alone, vulnerable, and completely exposed – Steve took a step in my direction while looking at me up and down from head to toe and said, "Oh yeah, you most definitely have potential!" No longer feeling safe and seeing him walking toward me, I ran out of his house while putting on my shirt, jumped on my bike, and raced home as fast as I could. That short bike ride home felt like the longest 10 minutes of my life. I was afraid and did not know what to do. I knew I had to tell an adult but I was afraid of my father's reaction. What would dad do? Would he do something that would lead to him going to jail or getting hurt? As a way of protecting my father, I never shared my experience with anyone, and I never saw Steve again. I repressed my traumatic experience, and it remained dormant for 20 years, until my patient awoke the little boy within me. He was finally heard after all these years.

My patient became a reflection of Steve, due to her attraction to teenage boys, a projection of my psyche that made it difficult for me to continue working with her. In a sense, I became the same little boy that ran away from Steve 20 years ago. I struggled through the last few months of therapy with this patient as termination approached due to funding issues within the program; however, during those sessions I constantly found myself doing the only thing I knew how to do: to run and run as hard as I could to protect the little boy within me. My life became even more difficult when my patient began to stalk me after termination. Her actions were constant reminders of my trauma and continued for a year after termination. I endured the situation alone because my clinical supervisor was no longer working for the program next door after it was closed due to funding issues with the county. In addition, my program did not have a clinical supervisor on staff and depended on the psychologist next door when in need of clinical assistance or guidance. I was left to defend myself in the same fashion I had 20 years prior – avoiding and compartmentalizing what was happening to me. Eventually, I was transferred to another program within the county, which was a relief. Although this was a very difficult time for me, I was able to overcome my struggles by finally facing Steve through personal therapy and also by reconnecting with my clinical supervisor shortly after he retired from the county.

Relevance of the Research for Clinical Psychology

Although there is vast literature on the topic of countertransference, a clear and universal definition continues to elude the field of psychology. Attempts to define the phenomenon vary largely according to theoretical orientation. The analyst's countertransference response within treatment, whether tied more to their internal world or the subjective experience of the patient, is an intricate part of treatment. However, the ways in which countertransference experiences are perceived and handled differ widely within the profession. Throughout my professional career, I have come to the understanding that strong, emotionally charged countertransference responses are commonplace. Unfortunately, such countertransference experiences are commonly "swept" under the rug as a way of ignoring the analyst's narcissistic wound and perceived failed attempts at remaining the objective and detached surgeon originally urged by Freud (1912/1953). The phenomenon of countertransference is then seen by many as impermissible, shameful, and possibly damaging to the profession as a whole (Sedgwick, 1994). This, however, is not necessarily true, as the perception of countertransference is interdependent on the analyst's theoretical perspective. Given that a transtheoretical definition of countertransference continues to circumvent the field of psychology, further exploration of the subject is necessary. Further investigation may assist analysts and therapists in gaining a greater and more comprehensive understanding of countertransference while also providing a positive conceptualization of the universality of the phenomenon. In addition, a universal understanding of countertransference would allow for a greater self-awareness and understanding of countertransference manifestations regardless of their origin. A greater understanding of countertransference will lead to a greater understanding of analysts' emotional response within treatment, and a greater understanding of themselves.

An Outline of the Book by Chapter

Before venturing into the world of countertransference, I would like to provide the reader with a few words on the content and organization of this book, including an explanation justifying why the writings of specific theorists were used and reviewed. In addition, I would like to provide the reader with some limitations to the book as a whole. Please keep in mind that although a robust sample of theoretical writings was selected for this book, not all theoretical perspectives were included. Influential psychologists such as James Hillman, Wilfred Bion, Marie-Louise von Franz, and Alfred Adler, to name a few, were not included. In addition, a qualitative approach, or more specifically, a philosophical hermeneutic inquiry, was used when examining the selected writings. Future research on countertransference would benefit from expanding on the foundation of this book by including additional theoretical approaches on the subject and integrating a quantitative point of view into the research. Limitations and recommendations will be discussed in further detail in Chapter 8.

Chapter 1 is an in-depth explanation of transference, including a review of its meaning and therapeutic use while also exploring how it can influence treatment and the therapeutic relationship. This chapter focuses specifically on the influential writings of Sigmund Freud and Melanie Klein since the concept was initially introduced by Freud and later expanded by Klein. Throughout the years, the writings of Freud and Klein continue to be foundational in the development and expansion of psychological concepts and ideas, with this situation being no different. The second part of the chapter will review more current writings on the subject while documenting the evolution of transference as a whole. Although this book focuses specifically on the phenomenon of countertransference, it becomes difficult to gain a thorough understanding of countertransference without having an understanding of transference. This chapter aims to provide the reader with that needed understanding.

Chapter 2 is a comprehensive analysis of countertransference from a depth psychological perspective. As part of this analysis, the psychological understandings of some of the most influential minds in psychoanalysis, such as Sigmund Freud, Melanie Klein, Donald Winnicott, Margaret Little, Heinrich Racker, and Lewis Aron, were examined. In order to provide a comprehensive analysis of countertransference, five distinct views on countertransference were presented, with each view representing an evolution of sorts and a change in the psychoanalytic understanding and approach to countertransference. This chapter also explores the importance of the analyst knowing themselves as a way of preventing their unresolved conflicts from interfering in treatment and instead using such wounds as a way of gaining a deeper understanding of the patient's woundedness, creating a unique push and pull dynamic that provides a view into the patient's psyche and ultimately facilitating healing.

Chapter 3 focuses on providing the reader with an in-depth analysis of countertransference in Jungian analysis. Although many books on countertransference tend to ignore the works of Carl Jung, his writings on the topic have been instrumental in gaining a deeper understanding of the phenomenon, especially since one of the main focal points of Jungian analysis is the use of countertransference. Similar to the Freudian view, the premise of Jungian analysis is the analysis and interpretation of the patient's transference; however, when combined with the analyst's countertransference experience, an interaction takes place between the patient and analyst, a push and pull between the transference and countertransference response of the therapeutic dyad that allows for a greater understanding of the patient. In addition, this chapter explores the interfering aspects of countertransference while also promoting the benefits of the analyst's personal analysis. The final third of the chapter provides a thorough description of the archetypal dimensions and manifestations of countertransference while also reviewing Jung's understanding of the unconscious, more specifically, understanding how the personal and collective unconscious affect countertransference responses and manifestations. Although many Jungian concepts were developed in the early to mid-1900s, Jung was ahead of his time, setting the path for many newer understandings of countertransference.

The primary focus of Chapter 4 is to examine the therapeutic benefits of countertransference dreams, including providing the reader with a thorough description and explanation of the role countertransference dreams play in treatment. The subject has been scarcely discussed because of the changing perceptions regarding its significance and prominence in analytic treatment, and the belief that such dreams are a disturbance within the analyst that can negatively impact treatment. In other words, countertransference dreams pose a threat of exposure to the analyst's own neurosis. As part of this review, the different types of countertransference dreams were categorized and reviewed while also highlighting the benefits of analyzing such dreams.

Chapter 5 discusses the significance of countertransference from a cognitive-behavioral approach. Since cognitive-behavioral therapy focuses on technical factors rather than relational ones, it is commonly assumed that countertransference has little therapeutic value or that it simply does not occur when using such treatment modality. This has paved the way for expanding the cognitive-behavioral understanding of countertransference and viewing it as a recurring phenomenon, resulting in more literature being written on the subject. One factor that may have resulted in the minimalization of countertransference within cognitive-behavioral therapy is semantics, as cognitive-behavioral theorists prefer using theory-specific language to separate countertransference from its psychodynamic origins. In addition, cognitive-behavioral therapy stresses the importance of material close to the surface and relatively close to the present, focusing on the here-and-now instead of influences from the patient's past. Cognitive-behavioral techniques are also considered to be more standardized and formulaic than other approaches, making the therapist's vulnerabilities and internal conflicts less relevant to treatment. This belief, however, has evolved over time, with a new school of thought emerging that stresses the importance of the therapist's role in treatment. This change has evolved to the point of exploring the origins of countertransference by discussing the role of schemas in countertransference reactions while also categorizing maladaptive schemas that influence the course of treatment. Although cognitive-behavioral literature continues to minimize the therapist's internal experience, it is essential to review the effect countertransference can have on treatment, especially with cognitive-behavioral therapy being one of the most commonly used treatment modalities.

Chapter 6 explores the humanistic view and approach to countertransference. Although there is an infrequent focus on the phenomenon of countertransference, that is not to say that a therapist's internal conflicts and vulnerabilities are irrelevant. The countertransference phenomenon is evident in the works of James Bugental, Betty Meador, Irvin Yalom, and Carl Rogers; however, instead of using the term countertransference, they use language-specific to humanistic psychology when describing the phenomenon. Countertransference, however, goes against the very building blocks of humanistic psychology and is counterintuitive to the basic tenets of humanistic theory. Humanistic psychology argues the goodness of human beings by nature which negates the negative qualities of the therapist, minimizing unresolved conflicts of the therapist commonly associated with countertransference. Since humanistic psychology does not consider the therapist's thoughts and feelings as countertransference distortions, countertransference becomes nonexistent and is superseded by the therapist's respect and connection with the patient. This concept, however, does not negate the fact that countertransference still occurs within humanistic treatment approaches. This is examined by highlighting the inevitability of countertransference within treatment and how it can impact the required authenticity of the therapist to promote change. In addition, this chapter discusses the six necessary conditions outlined by Rogers that must exist within a therapeutic relationship to promote change. When such conditions are not met, the therapist loses their ability to remain authentic and congruent, affecting their ability to provide the client with unconditional positive regard due to their own unresolved conflicts.

The primary focus of Chapter 7 is to provide the reader with an in-depth description of the development of a transtheoretical definition of countertransference through the unification of commonalities observed from the interpretation of various theoretical writings dealing with the phenomenon. During the interpretation process, additional points of inquiry emerged that exerted their own significance and required further exploration, such as countertransference dreams and somatic countertransference. In addition, this chapter reviews the transcendent function, or the analytic third, that serves as a platform or bridge for psychic interactions between the patient and the analyst to take place. Through the exploration and interpretation of countertransference writings, additional psychological concepts such as reflective countertransference and persecutory countertransference were developed and provided a thorough explanation for deciphering the difference between positive and pathological forms of countertransference and how to address them. This chapter also highlights the analysis of the analyst to address the analyst's susceptibility to countertransference. However, this is not necessarily related to the analyst's neurosis alone but also to the extensiveness of the analyst's unconsciousness, an unconscious realm co-created in conjunction with the patient. Although distinguishing between pathological and nonpathological countertransference responses is difficult, this chapter stresses the importance of the analyst accepting their own countertransference response while maintaining distance from the patient's experience. This leads to a cycle where analysts learn about themselves through psychic interactions, which helps them become more empathetic toward their patients while improving the quality of treatment.

The eighth and final chapter explores the benefits of developing a transtheoretical definition for the phenomenon of countertransference. Additionally, this chapter reviews the applications and benefits of countertransference to the field of psychology while also acknowledging the limitations of the current definition resulting from the fact that not all theoretical perspectives were covered. As a result, this chapter reviews recommendations moving forward on how to expand on the definition and understanding of countertransference while also making suggestions regarding future methodological considerations based on the current limitations. This chapter concludes by focusing on the underutilization of countertransference in treatment due to the lack of a standard transtheoretical definition. The hope is that such a definition will result in a therapeutic environment that promotes healing for patients and those we serve.

Definition of Terms

Countertransference is an inevitable and ubiquitous phenomenon, occurring in all clinical work, but has been mainly investigated in psychoanalytic orientations. As a result, a number of psychoanalytic terms will be defined for the reader in this section. Definitions were gathered from a number of different sources, including books, articles, and online sources.

Archetypes: "Primordial, structural elements of the human psyche" (Sharp, 1991, p. 27).

Cathexis: Freudian term used to express

> the idea of physical energy being lodged in or attaching to itself to mental structures or processes, somewhat on the analogy of an electric charge . . . the term refers to the sum of psychic energy, which occupies or invests objects or some particular channel.
>
> (Fodor & Gaynor, 1966, p. 23)

Depressive position:

> A mental constellation defined by Klein as central in the child's development, normally first experienced towards the middle of the first year of life. It is repeatedly revisited and redefined throughout early childhood, and intermittently throughout life. Central is the realisation of hateful feelings and phantasies about the loved object, prototypically the mother. Earlier there were felt to be two separate part-objects; ideal and loved; persecuting and hated. In this period the main anxiety concerned survival of the self. In the depressive position anxiety is also felt on behalf of the object.
>
> (Spillius, Milton, Garvey, Couve, & Steiner, 2011, p. 84)

Ego: "Part of a person's mental apparatus which develops gradually under the influence of environmental forces or the id to protect the organism against internal or external threats. . . . The main task of the ego is self-preservation the organism" (Wolman, 1989, p. 106).

Id: "The mass of unbound energies, both libidinal and aggressive, which constitute part of the unconscious and influence conscious actions by seeking discharge and immediate gratification in accordance with its governing influence, the pleasure principle" (Wolman, 1989, p. 170).

Introjection: The ego's attempt of integrating "a large part of the outside world and make it the object of unconscious phantasies" (Spillius et al., 2011, p. 63).

Libido: "Vital impulse or energy; often, sexual desire. Often this word is found in its adjectival form. 'Libidinal energy' is that which propels an 'object instinct' like sexual desire" (www.geneseo.edu/~easton/humanities/Freud.htm).

Paranoid-schizoid position:

> Refers to a constellation of anxieties, defences and internal and external object relations that Klein considers to be characteristic of the earliest months of an infant's life and to continue to a greater or lesser extent into childhood and adulthood. . . . The chief characteristic of the paranoid-schizoid position is the splitting of both self and object into good and bad, with at first little or no integration between them.
>
> (Spillius et al., 2011, p. 63)

Phantasy: "The psychic representation of instinct. Instinct itself is a biological entity and so phantasy is the psychic representation of one's biology" (Ogden, 1984, p. 501).

Projection: "To attribute certain states of mind to someone else, something of the ego is thus perceived as occurring in someone else" (Spillius et al., 2011, p. 454).

Splitting of an object: The concept

> in which the individual begins life with the developmentally essential task of achieving a binary split between the "good" and "bad" aspects of himself and his object in the "paranoid-schizoid" position; the individual also splits himself in other ways and then moves painfully on to the process of integration in the "depressive position."
>
> (Spillius et al., 2011, p. 491)

Superego: "An internal structure or part of the self that, as the internal authority, reflects on the self, makes judgements, exerts moral pressure and is the seat of conscious, guilt and self-esteem" (Spillius et al., 2011, p. 147).

1 Transference

When looking at the guiding principles of psychotherapy, the premise has remained the same throughout the years: the ability and willingness to know oneself. This, however, requires the difficult tasks of looking at one's own shadow material and accessing the deepest parts of our unconscious. Freud believed that the therapeutic task in psychotherapy was "one of bringing to the knowledge of the patient the unconscious repressed impulses existing in his mind and, to this end, of uncovering the resistances that oppose themselves to this extension of his knowledge about himself" (Freud, 1919/1953, p. 392). By bringing the patient's unconscious conflicts into consciousness, they become tangible, making it possible for a patient to work on them through an emotional relationship with the analyst. It is this emotional "bond" that makes way for the transference to make itself felt and present during treatment.

The phenomenon of transference was first introduced by Freud and is one of his significant contributions to psychoanalytic theory. Freud initially saw transference as an avenue to uncovering repressed traumatic memories; however, his view shifted as a result of a common theme he noted during analysis of his patients, in particular Dora, one of his most famous patients. During his analysis of Dora, Freud noted unconscious feelings and phantasies coming to the surface for Dora during treatment. To Freud what appeared to be feelings initially directed toward a person of importance from the patient's earlier life experiences were being transferred toward the analyst. Freud described the transference as follows:

> New editions or facsimiles of the impulses and phantasies . . . are aroused and made conscious during the progress of the analysis; but they have this peculiarity, which is characteristic for their species, that they replace some earlier person by the person of the physician. To put it another way: a whole series of psychological experiences are revived, not as belonging to the past, but as applying to the person of the physician at the present moment. Some of these transferences have a content which differs from that of their model in no respect whatever except for the substitution. These then – to keep to the same metaphor – are merely new impressions or reprints.

DOI: 10.4324/9781003320180-2

Others are more ingeniously constructed; their content has been subjected to a moderating influence – to *sublimation*, as I call it – and they may even become conscious, by cleverly taking advantage of some real peculiarity in the physician's person or circumstances and attaching themselves to that. These, then, will be no longer new impressions, but revised editions.

(Freud, 1905/1964, p. 116)

This led to a shift in Freud's view of transference. Although he saw transference as "the most powerful resistance to the treatment" (Freud, 1912/1958, p. 101) and an obstacle to psychoanalysis, he also saw it as a portal to the unconscious, allowing for a greater understanding of unconscious phantasies and innate drives. Through the psychotherapeutic relationship, transference elicits "new editions of the old conflicts" (Freud, 1917/1963, p. 454). The transfer of unconscious phantasies and impulses directed toward the analyst for the most part remained unchanged from the original experience; however, they occasionally take on an additional dimension of some sort, incorporating characteristics of the analyst. In other words, transference allows for the unification of the past with the present, allowing for the re-living of past experiences through the projection of unconscious phantasies aimed toward a new person. Transference thus becomes a distortion of reality brought on by innate drives and unmet libidinal needs, confusing the past with the present (Freud, 1912/1958). Freud (1912/1958) stated,

[t]he unconscious impulses do not want to be remembered in the way the treatment desires them to be, but endeavour to reproduce themselves in accordance with the timelessness of the unconscious and its capacity for hallucination. Just as happens in dreams, the patient regards the products of the awakening of his unconscious impulses as contemporaneous and real; he seeks to put his passions into action without taking any account of the real situation.

(Freud, 1912/1958, p. 108)

As a way of explaining the awakening of the patient's unconscious impulses, Freud focused on an individual's capacity to love.

According to Freud, a person's capacity to love is determined by their innate disposition and the influences brought on by early life experiences – the individual

has acquired a specific method of his own in his conduct of his erotic life – that is, in the preconditions to falling in love which he lays down, in the instincts he satisfies and the aims he sets himself in the course of it.

(Freud, 1912/1958, p. 99)

Through this interaction, an individual develops what Freud termed "stereotype plates," which serve as a script for future interactions with new objects that meet such stereotypes, allowing for the repetition, or re-living of past experiences. Portions of the stereotype are available to the conscious personality and remain in contact with reality. However, unmet *libidinal* impulses and erotic interests remain unconscious, living only in phantasy and remaining completely unconscious, away from reality, and unknown to the personality's conscious (Freud, 1912/1958). Unmet libidinal impulses are what motivate us to seek gratification from others. It is that need for love that causes a person to approach each new relationship or interaction with libidinal anticipatory notions created by conscious and unconscious libidinal impulses. Unsatisfied libidinal urges will search for others to latch on to, and in the case of analysis, the analyst becomes that object and target of libidinal *cathexis*, introducing them to a psychical "series" formed by the patient (Freud, 1912/1958). Freud stated,

> [t]he doctor tries to compel him to fit these emotional impulses into the nexus of the treatment and of his life-history, to submit them to intellectual consideration and to understand then in the light of their psychical value. This struggle between the doctor and the patient, between intellect and instinctual life, between understanding and seeking to act, is played out almost exclusively in the phenomena of transference.
>
> (Freud, 1912/1958, p. 108)

Transference is inevitable; however, it is not something caused by treatment: "It merely brings them to light, like so many other hidden psychical factors" (Freud, 1905/1964, p. 117). Freud added, "But it should not be forgotten that it is precisely they that do us the inestimable service of making the patient's hidden and forgotten erotic impulses immediate and manifest" (Freud, 1912/1958, p. 108). In addition, Freud argued that one of the most difficult tasks of treatment was the analyst's ability to manage the transference. However, he also stressed the important role the analyst plays in the manifestations of libidinal impulses and the uncovering of resistance within patients.

Through transference it becomes possible to work through the resistance of patients as they continue to re-live previous experiences in the here and now by influencing new experiences with elements of the past. The re-living or repeating of an experience is a defense to remembering, keeping libidinal wishes and desires unconscious. Instead of focusing on a particular problem or experience from the patient's past, the analyst concentrates on the present, what is currently being experienced by the patient, what is present in treatment, and what is being re-lived. The analyst will study "whatever is present for the time being on the surface of the patient's mind, and he employs the art of interpretation mainly for the purpose of recognizing the resistances which appear there, and making them conscious to the patient" (Freud, 1914/1958, p. 147). Through this reading of energy between patient and analyst, the analyst is able to expose the resistance unknown to the patient, bringing them to the forefront through interpretation and allowing the patient to make connections with the forgotten situations. The resistance is seen and treated as a present-day force while still tracing it back to its past origin. What the analyst does is "fill in the gaps in memory; dynamically speaking, it is to overcome resistance due to repression" (Freud, 1914/1958, p. 148). In other words, the analyst is finding the missing or lost pieces to a puzzle representing the patient's life experiences.

According to Freud (1914/1958), it is necessary and important to understand and interpret the patient's repetitive patterns and re-living of past experiences. Transference allows the analyst to follow the pull of unconscious libidinal impulses present during treatment and bring them to consciousness and reality. The psychical energy keeping these impulses unconscious now becomes the resistance to them becoming conscious (Freud, 1914/1958). Freud stated, "We may say that the patient does not remember anything of what he has forgotten and repressed, but acts it out. He reproduces it not as memory but as an action; he repeats it, without, of course, knowing that he is repeating it" (1914/1958, p. 150). In other words, the patient does not remember certain experiences or behaviors but instead acts toward the analyst in a way that reflects those behaviors and experiences, re-living and repeating the past, or "remembering" through repetition and acting out, occurring not only in treatment but also in other relationships within the patient's life (Freud, 1914/1958). Creating a container to "act out" is essential to treatment, providing the resistance and compulsion an arena to make itself present. Freud stated,

> [t]he main instrument, however, for curbing the patient's compulsion to repeat and for turning into a motive for remembering lies in the handling of the transference. We render the compulsion harmless, and indeed useful, by giving it the right to assert itself in a definitive field. We admit it into the transference as a playground in which it is allowed to expand in almost complete freedom and in which it is expected to display to us everything in the way of pathogenic instincts that is hidden in the patient's mind. . . . The transference thus creates an intermediate region between illness and real life through which the transition from the one to the other is made. The new condition has taken over all the features of the illness; but it represents an artificial illness which is at every point accessible to our intervention. It is a piece of real experience, but one which has been made possible by favourable conditions, and it is of a provisional nature. From the repetitive reactions which are exhibited in the transference we are led along the familiar path to the awakening of the memories, which appear without difficulty, as it were, after the resistance has been overcome.
>
> (pp. 154–155)

Once the resistance is uncovered by the analyst, the patient becomes acquainted with it, becoming aware of what has been hidden and repressed in the unconscious. Awareness of the resistance provides patients with a forum to familiarize themselves with it, making it possible to work through and overcome it regardless of its pull to prevent such. Once the resistance reaches its peak, the analyst is able to discover the repressed instinctual impulses that nourish and keep the resistance alive, making the patient aware of its existence and influence (Freud, 1914/1958). Although working through the resistance is considered a difficult task for the patient, it is a necessity that fosters the greatest change within the patient as "one cannot overcome an enemy who is absent or not within range" (Freud, 1914/1958, p. 152). Freud added,

> [t]he transference thus creates an intermediate region between illness and real life through which the transition from the one to the other is made. The new condition has taken over all the features of the illness; but it represents an artificial illness which is at every point accessible to our intervention from the repetitive reaction which are exhibited in the transference we are led along the familiar paths to the awakening of memories, which appear without difficulty, as it were, after the resistance has been overcome.
>
> (1914/1958, pp. 154–155)

Freud argued that by removing the resistance and bringing the transference into consciousness, the patient is able to conceptualize the issue at hand and move toward the goal of healing and gaining a deeper understanding of themself.

Although many followed after Freud and expanded the concept of transference, Melanie Klein greatly enhanced our understanding of transference and discussed the techniques used in comprehending the transference within analysis, specifically with her work with children. Like Freud, Klein (1952/1984) was of the belief that transference originated from birth through what she called object relations, an internal world organization of early versions of one's experience of others, influencing all human interactions and one's experience of the world. Through analysis, the patient is able to transfer these experiences and emotions forming one's character onto the analyst, resulting in the activation of unresolved conflicts. This transference leads to the patient's use of repeated defense mechanisms to deal with conflicts and anxieties. For Klein, the deeper into the unconscious and the further back the analyst can go into the patient's past, the better the understanding of the transference.

According to Klein (1952/1984), from birth the infant develops an anxiety *persecutory* in nature and has destructive impulses toward an object, usually a parent, raising the fear of retaliation by the object, or the fear of its own destruction and annihilation which she linked to the infant's death instinct. This anxiety is heightened by external experiences of the object, arising from frustration and discomfort during its earliest days of life. It is the infant's experience of birth and of a new and unknown environment that gives rise to some of these terrors. The initial comforting experiences by an object, usually the mother, after birth are deemed as good by the infant due to the object's ability to remove pain, discomfort, frustration, and confusion. It is this experience that leads to the initial *splitting of an object*. The feelings of love, admiration, and gratification are directed toward the "good" breast, while persecutory anxieties are aimed toward the "bad" breast. In other words, the good breast is seen as the protector and the source of love while the bad breast is considered to be the source of persecution, leading to the infant aiming its rage and hatred toward the breast. Since the infant cannot decipher between a whole or split object, it keeps the good and bad breast apart from each other as two separate entities. The infant reaches a sense of safety and security through its relationship with the good breast, transforming it into its protector against its persecutory counterpart, the bad breast. At this primitive level of experience, the good breast is hypothesized as being the ideal and omnipotent protector against the bad breast or object of persecution. Klein termed this early splitting between good and bad and its attendant anxieties resulting from such process *the paranoid-schizoid position* (Klein, 1952/1984).

Object relations are initiated through *projection* and *introjection* as they are linked with the emotions and anxieties of the infant. According to Klein (1952/1984), "by projecting, i.e., deflecting libido and aggression on to the mother's breast, the basis for object-relations is established: by introjecting the object, first of all the breast, relations to internal objects come into being" (p. 49). It is through the introjection of the breast that formation of the *superego* begins, making the core of the superego both the good and bad breast. Through the processes of projection and introjection, the internal and external interact, leading to the fluctuation between reality and phantasy, between love and hate, leading to "an interplay between persecutory anxiety and idealization – both referring to internal and external objects; the idealized object being a corollary of the persecutory, extremely bad one" (Klein, p. 50).

As the ego matures and continues to develop, it gains the capacity for synthesis and integration, which leads to the development of a new kind of anxiety that Klein named depressive anxiety, resulting in the advent of the *depressive position*. The infant begins to believe that its aggressive impulses toward the "bad breast" are now a danger to the "good breast," with the anxiety being reinforced as the infant began to introject and see the mother as a whole person. The aggressive impulses are believed in phantasy to have destroyed or are destroying the whole object based on the infant's greed and uncontainable hostility. The infant begins to see these aggressive impulses being aimed at a loved person. To Klein, these anxieties and defenses are related to the loss and destruction of loved internal and external objects (Klein, 1952/1984). Klein stated,

> [t]he analysis of very young children has taught me that there is no instinctual urge, no anxiety, situation, no mental process which does not involve objects, external or internal; in other words, object-relations are at the *centre* of emotional life. Furthermore, love and hatred, phantasies, anxieties, and defenses are also operative from the beginning and are *ab initio* indivisibly linked with object-relations.

> (Klein, 1952/1984, p. 53)

With object relations being at the center of emotional life, the infant's anxiety over the destruction of the good breast through their aggressive impulses toward the bad breast, the infant is showing the ability to see the mother as a whole object instead of the previously split good and bad object. This symbolizes the beginning of integrated object relations within the infant.

According to Klein (1952/1984), transference and object relations develop in the same manner, requiring the need to analyze internal and external objects prominent during early infancy as these prototype relationships established during infancy form an individual's character and are the basis of one's experience of the outer world and others. By doing so we can

> [f]ully appreciate the interconnection between positive and negative transference only if we explore the early interplay between love and hate, and the vicious circle of aggression, anxieties feelings of guilt and increased aggression, as well as the various aspects of objects towards whom these conflicting emotions and anxieties are directed.
>
> (Klein, 1952/1984, p. 53)

During infancy there are few people involved in the life of the child; however, their perception signifies multiple objects as they appear to the child in different aspects, both the good and bad of the object, resulting in the splitting of the object, and eventual development of positive and negative transference. However, through the negative transference we can access the deeper levels of the patient's unconscious, with the key, according to Klein, being the analysis of the interconnection between positive and negative transferences (Klein, 1952/1984). Through transference the analyst plays a number of different roles, including that of a parent, or a portion of the id, ego, or superego of the patient. Understanding early object relations grants the analyst information related to the various roles exhibited and projected by the patient during treatment. However, it is necessary to identify which portion of the object or self is being recharged and transferred to the analyst at any given moment. During infancy, the image of the parent or object becomes distorted because of the child's projection and internalization of it, with the current love object being a representation, or imago, of the original object. Concurrently, a substantial portion of the object is preserved in its *phantastic nature*. For the infant, every external experience is interconnected with phantasy, whereas all phantasies share components of an actual experience. By analyzing the transference at its depths, it becomes possible to uncover the past and understand the fantasy and reality aspects of it, with the strength of the transference determined by the origin of interchanges between phantasy and reality (Klein, 1952/1984). This is known as psychic reality, the amalgamation of actual reality and an individual's inner world experience of it.

Transference in general is seen as a direct reference to the analyst in relation to the patient's psychological material. By deducing the unconscious elements originated during infancy from the transference experienced in the "here and now," the analyst gains an understanding of the functioning of the ego as well as the defenses against the anxieties present within the transference. When presented with a similar situation, or the re-living of a similar experience, the patient is expected to respond and deal with the anxieties in a similar fashion as they did previously. The patient will

> turn away from the analyst as he attempted to turn away from his primal objects; he tries to split the relations to him, keeping him either as a good or as a bad figure: he deflects some of the feelings and attitudes experienced towards the analyst on to other people in his current life, and this is part of his "acting out."
>
> (Klein, 1952/1984, pp. 55–56)

With transference being rooted in early object relations, allowing the reenactment or re-living of the patient's experience through the use of the analyst provides the analyst with a greater understanding of the patient's defenses and unconscious material.

According to Klein (1952/1984), early object relations are the foundation for understanding transference; however, this does not minimize the importance or need to analyze the emotional development brought on by later object relations, covering "all that lies between the current situation and the earliest experiences" (p. 56). In fact, Klein felt it was impossible to access early emotions and object relations without understanding the patient's later developments and outside experiences. Through the interrelatedness of early and later experiences, it is possible to connect the past and present of the patient's mind. By integrating the patient's mind as a whole, the need for defenses (i.e., splitting and repression) diminishes, and the ego strengthens. Unconscious phantasies are integrated with the ego, leading to an enhancement and strengthening of the patient's personality while also revising early object relations. This also leads to the deduction of the compulsive need to repeat previous experiences brought on by persecution resulting from primitive defense mechanisms such as splitting and projection, and the guilt associated with the depressive position and the patient's concern for the well-being of their objects. Per Klein, these changes are only possible through the analysis of transference, and by linking them to the earliest object relations and how they manifest in the patient's current life and their vision of the analyst.

More recent perspectives on transference attempt to expand on the views of Freud and Klein. In the case of Otto Kernberg (1992), he attempted to bridge the gap between the Freudian drive model and the emphasis Klein placed on the first year of life. Kernberg believed that

> affects from their very origin have a cognitive aspect, that they contain at least an appraisal of the "goodness" or "badness" of the immediate perceptive constellation, and that this appraisal . . . determines a felt motivation for action either towards or away from a certain stimulus or situation.
>
> (pp. 5–6)

Building on this idea, Kernberg argued that affects were "the psychobiological building blocks of drives and the earliest motivational systems" (p. 8). Such an approach challenged our understanding and belief that erotogenic zones were the primary source of libido, instead arguing that libido should be considered all "physiologically activated functions and bodily zones that become involved in affectively invested interactions" between infant and mother (p. 9). As a result, a shift occurred that placed the focus on social functions and role reenactments instead of bodily functions. In other words, internalized object relations are responsible for energizing the physiological zones. This concept allowed for the input of new affective experiences throughout an individual's life, resulting in the organization of libidinal and aggressive drives and a hierarchical motivational system. If a specific drive is activated through an intrapsychic conflict, the corresponding affects would be activated in addition to the activation brought on by an internalized object relation connected to an object representation or affective state. Therefore, affects become representations of an individual's drives.

Kernberg (1992) emphasized the analysis of transference and believed it consisted of analyzing the activation of internalized object relations in the here-and-now. This process also includes analyzing id, ego, and superego structures in addition to intrastructural and interstructural conflicts. For Kernberg, internalized object relations are not necessarily representations of the past but instead "a combination of realistic and fantasied-and often highly distorted-internalizations of such past object relations and defenses against them under the effects of instinctual drive derivatives" (p. 103). Although transference analysis aims to analyze the activation of internalized object relations in the here-and-now, a tension exists between the here-and-now and the unconscious genetic determinants of the patient's developmental history. As a result, Kernberg argued that transference manifestations presented themselves as "instinctual impulses expressed as affects" or "identifications reflecting internalized object relations" that provide a frame of reference to the metapsychological understanding of the unconscious and how it presents itself in consciousness (p. 104).

According to Kernberg (1992), transference manifestations are characterized by distorted unconscious representations of the patient's conflict with an internalized object from their past. These manifestations become distorted through defenses such as repression and splitting and function in keeping the experience unconscious. To bring the unconscious transference meaning to the here-and-now, Kernberg suggested the use of interpretation as the first means to understand the relationship between the unconscious present and the unconscious past. In addition, instead of attempting to connect conscious and preconscious states related to the patient's experience of the analyst with the patient's conscious and unconscious past, Kernberg suggested using the patient's free associations to uncover the unconscious meaning of the patient's transference in the here-and-now. As a result, the patient's unconscious past is reviled in the form of past internalized object relations being superimposed onto the analyst.

Although Kernberg emphasized the analysis of transference and the use of interpretation, he warned against developing premature assumptions of genetic origins and unconscious transference meanings (Kernberg, 1992). Kernberg (1993) stated, "A theoretical frame that locates the patient's dominant conflicts in a predetermined area or time seems to me to restrict both the analyst's and the patient's freedom to explore the origins of the unconscious present in the unconscious past" (p. 105). Since Kernberg believed that activating internalized object relations would eventually uncover their origin and meaning, he discouraged committing to hypotheticals and instead encouraged the patient's free association, which would allow them to explore the unconscious meaning of their behaviors in the here-and-now. Once the object relation in the transference becomes conscious, the analyst can work toward reconstructing the patient's past, leading to the interpretation and consideration of genetic determinants activated by the patient's experience of unconscious intrapsychic conflict in the here-and-now.

Lewis Aron (1991, 1996) and Owen Renik (1999) continued to redefine the concept of transference by adopting a relational view of the phenomenon and focusing on the analyst's subjectivity within treatment. Aron (1993) emphasized the intersubjective experience between the therapeutic dyad and believed the therapeutic process was heavily influenced by the relationship and interactions of the patient and analyst. Analysis was seen as a two-person psychology and a co-constructed phenomenon. Renik (1999), on the other hand, believed that an analyst's individual psychology, their past, personality, and countertransference experiences were unavoidable, playing an essential role in treatment. In Chapter 2, the relational view of transference/countertransference will be discussed in further detail.

Westen and Gabbard (2002) further expanded on the work of Aron and Renik and added some additional wrinkles to their conceptualization of transference. Like Aron and Renik, Westen and Gabbard emphasized the analyst's subjectivity within treatment. Westen and Gabbard stated:

> The analyst's subjectivity and personal characteristics cannot be eliminated with a mask of anonymity. . . . There is now a broad consensus that the analyst is always a participant in the analytic interaction, and the way the analyst participates influences the patient's transferences.
>
> (p. 120)

As a result, Westen and Gabbard argued against the notion of the blank-screen analyst. Although the role of the blank-screen analyst was to prevent the "contamination" of the transference, it is essential to remember that the analytic situation and the characteristics of the analyst will activate certain transferences while inhibiting others. Blank-screen analyst or not, the analyst will continuously influence the patient's transference. Westen and Gabbard also viewed transference as more than a defense or the displacement of libidinal energy or the activation of internalized object relations, and instead as a "continual construction and reconstruction of thoughts, feelings, wishes, fears, patterns of relating, and ways of regulating affect in the context of new relationship experiences that can be understood only in the context of old ones" (p. 130). In other words, transference represents the integration of past and present experiences, allowing the analyst to see how the patient interacts and responds under certain circumstances within treatment.

According to Westen and Gabbard (2002), several misconceptions exist related to treatment and transference. Resolving the patient's transference does mean the patient should terminate treatment since patients experience multiple transferences and not simply just one. These transferences are continuous and frequently changing and are activated throughout treatment based on different aspects of the analyst and the analytical situation. In addition, these transferences reflect the various psychological processes and transference paradigms of the patient.

Although Westen and Gabbert highlighted the benefits of transference analysis, they cautioned against the expectation that a patient's most important dynamic will present itself in the transference. They also discouraged the expectation that what presents itself in treatment will always be of therapeutic value. This, however, does not devalue a patient's transference experience. Transference reactions, regardless of their origin, are "likely to shed substantial light on important relational configurations, defenses, and conflicts, because the analytic situation inherently activates certain kinds of relationship paradigms (such as those related to authority, attachment, and intimacy)" (Westen & Gabbard, 2002, p. 129). This experience provides the analyst with a firsthand experience of how the patient responds and interacts with others.

2 Countertransference From a Depth Psychological Perspective

According to Epstein and Feiner (1988), Natterson (1991), and Gelso and Hayes (2007), the psychodynamic view of countertransference has evolved over time and resulted in a number of different perspectives on the phenomenon. Epstein and Feiner (1988) described the three different psychodynamic perspectives of countertransference in the following fashion:

1. Classical conception: "Countertransference is viewed as the unconscious resistive reaction of the analyst to the transference of the patient, or part of the patient, and as containing both neurotic and nonneurotic elements" (p. 293). When mentioning nonneurotic elements of countertransference, Epstein and Feiner (1988) are referring to the nonpathological response on behalf of the analyst.
2. Totalistic conception: Countertransference is comprised of all feelings and attitudes of the therapist toward the patient.
3. Complementary conception: Countertransference is viewed "as the natural, role-responsive, necessary complement of counterpart to the transference of the patient, or to his style of relatedness" (Epstein & Feiner, 1988. p. 293).

Unlike Epstein and Feiner (1988), Natterson (1991) does not see views on countertransference as differing perspectives, but instead as simply the evolution of the phenomenon. According to Natterson (1991),

> The evolution of countertransference has occurred in three important steps: countertransference as:
>
> 1. Disruptive, destructive, with its detection and elimination being necessary to relieve blockage of the therapy,
> 2. Neurotic and potentially damaging if not analyzed and eliminated (or reduced); but often providing the therapeutic understanding of basic importance, thereby adding greatly to the progress of therapy,
> 3. A normative phenomenon; every therapist has abundant idiosyncratic responses to every patient, which play a fundamental part in the shape and course of the therapeutic events. (pp. 74–75)

DOI: 10.4324/9781003320180-3

Gelso and Hayes (2007) described the different perspectives of countertransference similar to Epstein and Feiner (1988); however, their description includes four different viewpoints, and a fifth based on their research and clinical experience:

1. The Classical View: "Countertransference is conceptualized as the therapist's largely unconscious, conflict-based reactions to the patient's transference. In this sense, countertransference may be seen as the therapist's transference to the patient's transference" (Gelso & Hayes, 2007, p. 5).
2. The Totalistic View: Countertransference is conceptualized as all of the therapist's attitudes and feelings towards the patient. . . . In other words, what the therapist feels at a given moment may well reveal what the patient is pulling for or is experiencing within the transference (Gelso & Hayes, 2007, p. 7).
3. The Complementary View: Countertransference is conceptualized as a complement or counterpart to the patient's transference or style of relating. The complementary view shares with the totalistic view the belief that the therapists' reactions (at least internal ones) are often inevitable, given the patient's defenses and ways of relating. The distinctiveness of this complementary conception resides in its articulation of the psychological dance that often carries out between therapist and patient. Each constantly affects and influences both internal and external reactions in the other, and the circle continues throughout treatment. Patients consciously or unconsciously "pull" for certain reactions in their therapists, and therapists experience the impulse to respond to their patients and so forth (Gelso & Hayes, 2007, pp. 9–10).
4. The Relational View: The relational view of countertransference shares a number of commonalities with the complementary view and tends to focus on the analyst's contribution and interactive nature of the phenomenon. Countertransference is conceptualized as the inevitable interaction of the patient's dynamics (his or her transference, realistic expression, personality, etc.) and the therapist's dynamics (unresolved conflicts, personality, needs, realistic expression). Countertransference is a co-construction between the therapist and the patient within the therapeutic hour (Gelso & Hayes, 2007, pp. 11–12).
5. Integrative View: The integrative view of countertransference is a conception that consists of elements of the four previously described views.

Although many contributed to the evolution of countertransference from a psychodynamic standpoint, this chapter will focus mainly on those who revolutionized the concept through the viewpoints described by Gelso and Hayes (2007).

Classical View

Sigmund Freud

The concept of countertransference was first introduced by Sigmund Freud in 1910; however, Freud was very contradictory in his message, leaving an uncertain perspective regarding the subject, an ambivalence that still remains today. Initially, Freud (1910/1953) warned against countertransference, considering it a hindrance to treatment. Freud stated:

> We have begun to consider the 'counter-transference', which arises in the physician as a result of the patient's influence on his unconscious feelings, and have nearly come to the point of requiring the physician to recognize and overcome this counter-transference in himself. Now that a larger number of people have come to practise psycho-analysis and mutually exchange their experiences, we have noticed that every analyst's achievement is limited by what his own complexes and resistances permit, and consequently we require that he should begin his practice with a self-analysis and should extend and deepen this constantly while making his observations on his patients. Anyone who cannot succeed in this self-analysis may without more ado regard himself as unable to treat neurotics by analysis.
>
> (p. 289)

As a result, Freud argued, nothing of worth could come from countertransference, believing that analysts should submit to self-analysis in order to work through their unresolved complexes and resistances. The inability to work through their neurosis would prevent analysts from working with and analyzing others (Lia, 2017). The purpose and focus of self-analysis was a preventive measure to control the analyst's complexes and resistances triggered by the patient. By ignoring the analyst's neurosis, countertransference became a barrier and a hindrance to treatment, negatively impacting the effects on the patient and on treatment.

Based on his understanding of countertransference at the time, Freud urged his colleagues to follow the model of a surgeon, stating,

> I cannot recommend my colleagues emphatically enough to take as a model in psycho-analytic treatment the surgeon who puts aside all his own feelings, including that of human sympathy, and concentrates his mind on one single purpose, that of performing the operation as skillfully as possible.
>
> (Freud, 1912/1953, p. 327)

Freud explained that it was not only necessary for analysts to eliminate their countertransference but also their personal feelings, in order to be effective within treatment. However, Freud added a new layer to his understanding of countertransference, resulting in a sense of confusion concerning the subject.

In 1912, Freud urged others to study themselves and their reactions to patients as a way of gaining a greater awareness of their unconscious, eventually leading to a greater understanding of the internal world of the patient. Through this dissection of the self, there can be a deeper understanding of the patient (Gelso & Hayes, 2007). Freud (1912/1953) stated:

> All these rules which I have brought forward coincide at one point which is easily discernible. They all aim at creating for the physician a complement to the "fundamental rule of psycho-analysis" for the patient. Just as the patient must relate all that self-observation can detect, and must restrain all the logical and affective objections which would urge him to select, so the physician must put himself in a position to use all that is told him for the purpose of interpretation and recognition of what is hidden in the unconscious, without substituting a censorship of his own for the selection which the patient forgoes. Expressed in a formula, he must bend his own unconscious like a receptive organ toward the emerging unconscious of the patient, be as a receiver of the telephone to the disc. As the receiver transmutes the electric vibrations included by the sound-waves back again into sound-waves, so is the physician's unconscious mind able to reconstruct the patient's unconscious, which has directed his associations, for the communications derived from it.
>
> (p. 328)

In other words, Freud argued, it was essential for analysts to know themselves and to use this understanding as a guiding principle to understand others. Self-analysis was no longer seen as a preventative measure and way of exploring and controlling the analyst's complexes and resistances, but instead as a way of bridging the patient and analyst by allowing the analyst a greater understanding of the patient through the use of an understanding of themselves.

Although Freud considered countertransference to be clinically significant, his contributions to the concept were never fully formed; he only wrote a total of four times on the subject (Gelso & Hayes, 2007). In addition, Freud's contradictory messages left much to be desired, leaving a trail of ambivalence and confusion. On the one hand, Freud encouraged analysts to gain a greater understanding of themselves and to use this newfound insight into treatment, while on the other, he was asking analysts to eliminate their countertransference reactions and personal feelings.

Melanie Klein

Within the field of psychoanalysis, one of the most influential minds continues to be that of Melanie Klein, who developed the theory of object relations. Klein, however, did not consider countertransference to be clinically useful, arguing that it was a neurotic response resulting from the analyst's unmet libidinal needs, a perception similar to the Freudian conceptualization of countertransference.

Klein considered countertransference to be nothing more than a disturbance to the analytic work, providing no therapeutic benefit to treatment and recommended against its use within treatment (Segal, 1992; Lia, 2017). In addition, countertransference also influences the analyst's technique within treatment, in particular in situations where patients are seeking reassurance in the form of love and affection as a result of their distress and anxiety (Klein, 1957/1984). The analyst's feelings and emotional responses toward the patient should always be treated as the analyst's pathology, and as such, require further analysis. In other words, countertransference serves as an obstacle to the exploration of the analyst's neurosis and unmet libidinal drives (Segal, 1992).

Although Klein warned against the hindrance of countertransference, her theoretical contributions, in particular, that of projective identification, provided the theoretical foundation for understanding and interpreting the analyst's emotional responses (Scharff & Scharff, 1998). In other words, as a result of Klein's work, countertransference is seen as a way for the analyst to identify with and understand the internal world of the patient, as it is "a state of mind induced in the analyst as a result of verbal and non-verbal actions by the patient, thus giving effect to the patient's phantasy of projective identification" (Spillius, 1988, p. 11). Although projective identification is a form of transference, it is being discussed in this chapter as a result of its influence on the furthering of countertransference, in particular, by the writings of Klein's understudies.

Klein introduced the concept of projective identification in 1946 as a result of her work with children. According to Scharff and Scharff (1998), Klein defined projective identification as the splitting of the unwanted or bad portion of the self or internal object and projecting it into an external object. In another instance, the patient will project the good part of the object into the analyst to ensure its preservation. In the case of analysis, the projection is made by the analyst in phantasy. The patient then begins to identify the projected part of the self/object with the external object. The projection no longer is felt to belong to the patient but instead is felt to be owned by the analyst. As a result of the projection, the analyst introjects and identifies with the projection and is momentarily controlled by the projected elements of the patient. The analyst may identify with the projected part and feel or act in a way that lives out the identification. Part of the analyst's task is to realize this, metabolize the projection, and return it to the patient in a way that can be tolerated and gradually integrated (Scharff & Scharff, 1998). In other words, through projective identification the patient is able to unconsciously communicate their state of mind with the analyst, eventually evoking the patient's state of mind within the analyst through the introjection of the patient's projection. This in turn is the transference/countertransference dynamic that takes place within analysis. Through the analyst's countertransference experience (i.e., identifying with the patient's internal world), the interpretation of the patient's transference becomes possible, which also fosters the possibility of psychic change within the patient (Scharff & Scharff, 1998).

Annie Reich

Like many of Freud's predecessors, Annie Reich (1951/1990) remained consistent with Freud's view of countertransference and was adamant in believing it had no therapeutic benefit to treatment, either as a way of understanding the patient or as a form of communicating therapeutically. According to Reich (1951/1990), countertransference is the unconscious conflict-based response of the analyst triggered by the patient's transference. Because the conflict within the analyst is based on early childhood experiences, the patient becomes a reflection and projection of the analyst's past, clouding the analyst's judgment and distorting the analyst's perception of the patient. Reich (1951/1990) argued that countertransference comprised

> [t]he effects of the analyst's own unconscious needs and conflicts on his understanding or technique. In such cases the patient represents for the analyst an object of the past on to whom past feelings and wishes are projected, just as it happens in the patient's transference situation with the analyst. The provoking factor for such an occurrence may be something in the patient's personality or material or something in the analytic situation as such. This is counter-transference in the proper sense.
>
> (p. 154)

The analyst's neurosis is seen through unresolved conflicts that become a barrier to treatment and a hindrance to the healing and psychological advancement of the patient. This occurrence becomes possible as the patient becomes a projection of the analyst's past while providing an arena in which the analyst acts out and re-experiences their neurosis as a result of their unresolved conflicts. In other words, the analyst's emotional response and countertransference manifestation become "a substitute for empathy" (Reich, 1960). In addition, the analyst's emotional response disregards what Reich felt was Freud's goal of analysis: analyzing ego pathology. Instead, countertransference focuses on influencing the object relations associated with the primitive needs of the id, ignoring the fact that "where id was, ego shall be" (Freud, 1933/1964, p. 80). Therefore, the analyst's emotional response prevents the psychological growth and healing of the patient while also preventing the development of the self. Countertransference then becomes an avenue for the analyst to act out and alleviate feelings of guilt and anxiety associated with the analyst's past (Reich, 1951/1990).

For Reich, the use of the analyst's emotional response in the form of countertransference removes the analyst from the necessary objectivity and analytic neutrality required in treatment. The expectation of the analyst is to refrain from having any sort of emotional response associated with the patient. Hence, experiencing a strong emotional cathexis to the patient becomes counterproductive, as it signals residual pathology related to the analyst's unresolved issues and can only be a result of such (Reich, 1960). Reich (1960) stated, "A neutralized cathexis of the patient is never relinquished. Thus, the analyst never loses sight of the patient as a separate being and at no time feels his own identity changed. This enables him to remain uninvolved" (p. 391). In such a fashion, countertransference is not a useful therapeutic tool; however, "the readiness to acknowledge its existence and the ability to overcome it is" (Epstein & Feiner, 1988, p. 292).

Although Reich did not believe in the therapeutic benefit of countertransference in and of itself, she deemed it a necessity of treatment. The lack of countertransference pointed toward the lack of interest by the analyst, which in turn is a source of countertransference (Reich, 1951/1990). Countertransference is a part of treatment; however, it should remain in the shadows of treatment instead of the forefront.

Totalistic View

Unlike the classical view of countertransference that considered countertransference a hindrance to treatment and of no therapeutic value, the totalistic view saw it as a useful tool to assist the analyst in gaining a greater understanding of the patient. The totalistic position considered countertransference as all attitudes and views by the analyst toward the patient (Epstein & Feiner, 1988; Gelso & Hayes, 2007). This perspective provided a different opinion on countertransference: instead of avoiding it, this perspective legitimized it by encouraging the analysis and understanding of it. This view began to gain popularity within psychoanalysis and required the analyst to reflect on their internal and external reactions to the patient. By analyzing their response to the patient, it became possible for the analyst to gain a greater understanding of the patient, their impact on others, and their internal world (Gelso & Hayes, 2007).

Donald Winnicott

Donald Winnicott (1994) was one of the first to effectively challenge the classical view of countertransference. Countertransference was not just the emotional response of the analyst triggered by the patient but also the psychological burden placed on the analyst resulting in hate toward the patient (Winnicott, 1994; Habibi-Kohlen, 2018). Winnicott described countertransference in the following fashion:

1. Abnormality in countertransference feelings, and set relationships and identifications that are under repression in the analyst. The comment on this is that the analyst needs more analysis, and we believe this is less of an issue among psychoanalysts than among psychotherapists in general.
2. The identifications and tendencies belonging to an analyst's personal experiences and personal development which provide the positive setting for his analytic work and make his work different in quality from that of any other analyst.

3. From these two I distinguish the truly objective countertransference, or if this is difficult, the analyst's love and hate in reaction to the actual personality and behaviour of the patient, based on objective observation. (p. 350)

In other words, there are a number of key components to analysis, including an objective frame of mind by the analyst to everything the patient brings to treatment. As a result, Winnicott (1994) emphasized the analysis of the analyst's repressed feelings, including their primitive aspects, to prevent the derailment of treatment. However, the treatment of patients can become an extension of this, as it becomes "an attempt on the part of an analyst to carry the work of his own analysis further than the point to which his own analyst could get him" (Winnicott, 1994, p. 351).

In addition, Winnicott (1994) also stressed the importance of studying the analyst's countertransference response, in particular, what he called the analyst's objective reaction to the patient, which includes the unavoidable love/hate response of the analyst toward the patient. The love/hate reactions of the analyst within the therapeutic relationship are related to the revelation of the patient's personality and behaviors brought on by the analyst's objective observations of the patient (Langs, 1976). Through the analyst's ability to hate the patient objectively, the patient is able to be objectively loved (Winnicott, 1994). This in turn brings us back to the analysis of the analyst. By going through their own analysis, analysts rid themselves of the "vast reservoirs of unconscious hate belonging to the past and to inner conflict" (Winnicott, 1994, p. 351).

To address hate in the countertransference, analysts place themselves in a role similar to that of the patient's mother at the time of the patient's infancy. In the same fashion as the mother tolerates her hate toward her child, the analyst is expected to tolerate hate for the patient (Winnicott, 1994). The mother tolerates the pain caused by her child without retaliation, just as the analyst tolerates pain caused by the patient (i.e., the burden of treatment). The mother tolerates the feelings of hate toward her child with the expectation of delayed gratification from the child. Similarly, the analyst often delays making the patient aware of their disdain for them until later in treatment. A sentimental environment prevents the patient from understanding the extent of their own hate. The patient needs hate to understand hate, and the analyst's hate toward the patient allows the patient to hate the analyst in return, granting the possibility of identifying with the analyst. By experiencing objective hate, the patient can experience objective love (Winnicott, 1994).

Winnicott (1988) expanded his description of countertransference as "the neurotic features that spoil the professional attitude and disturb the course of the analytic process" (p. 266). For instance, Winnicott warned against the analyst's pathological manifestations brought on by the countertransference responses triggered by the patient. The strengthening of the analyst's ego through personal analysis would prevent such disturbances; however, it is important for the analyst to remain vulnerable, as any changes in the structures of ego defenses would lessen the analyst's ability in dealing with new situations brought on by future patients (Winnicott, 1988).

Due to Winnicott's contributions, the countertransference views of classical analysis were challenged. Winnicott emphasized the therapeutic importance and benefits of countertransference and considered it not only as a source of information regarding the patient but of analysis as well. However, he maintained the classical belief that required the detoxification of the analyst through analysis.

Paula Heimann

Paula Heimann (1950), like Winnicott, challenged the classical view of countertransference that considered all countertransference reactions as a hindrance to treatment and a source of "trouble." Heimann argued against the notion of the "detached analyst" brought on by the belief that a well-trained analyst does not feel anything more than a sense of benevolence toward the patient, a concept similar to that of Freud's detached surgeon (Heimann, 1950). Heimann viewed countertransference, similar to transference in that it was not easy to simply separate and categorize the countertransference reactions of the analyst as those caused by unresolved issues of the analyst (parental projections) versus those brought on by the patient. The transference/countertransference dynamic within treatment is the result of a relationship between two individuals, the patient and analyst, and the nurturing and growth of the relationship allows for an emotional response on behalf of the analyst. Countertransference is more than simply transference on the part of the analyst; it is part of the analytic relationship, a creation of the patient and a part of their personality. As a result, Heimann defined countertransference as all feelings the analyst felt toward the patient (Heimann, 1950).

Heimann rejected the negative and popular views of countertransference of the day and instead focused on the advancement of analysis through the use of countertransference responses (Epstein & Feiner, 1988). According to Heimann, countertransference provides an avenue in which the analyst can make interpretations not just from an intellectual standpoint but also from an emotional one based on the feelings activated within the analyst during treatment. The analyst becomes a reflection of the patient and the emotional response is in relation to the patient's unconscious, making it an important tool within analysis and "an instrument of research into the patient's unconscious" (Heimann, 1950, para. 7). Heimann, however, warned against the mishandling of countertransference because of the pathological and nonpathological reactions of the analyst. Like her predecessors, Heimann stressed the importance of the analysis of the analyst, believing the lack of analysis resulted in poor interpretations on behalf of the analyst (Heimann, 1950). The successful analyst requires emotional stability in order to follow the emotional responses and unconscious phantasies of the patient. Such emotional stability provides the analyst the ability to follow the patient's associations in conjunction with their own emotional response. Heimann (1950) stated:

> Our basic assumption is that the analyst's unconscious understands that of his patient. This rapport on the deep level comes to the surface in the form of feelings which the analyst notices in response to his patient, in his 'counter-transference'. This is the most dynamic way in which his patient's voice reaches him. In the comparison of feelings roused in himself with his patient's associations and behaviour, the analyst possesses a most valuable means of checking whether he has understood or failed to understand his patient. . . . Therefore the analyst's emotional sensitivity needs to be extensive rather than intensive, differentiating and mobile.
>
> (para. 11)

The lack of emotional stability prevents analysts from seeing their emotional response as problematic, because they are in accordance with the meaning and perception they are interpreting and understanding. Analysts who have not processed their own infantile conflicts and anxieties will project onto their patients what rightfully belongs to them. As a result, the analyst's reasoning becomes clouded by the emotions brought on by their neurosis. In other words, "the analyst's unconscious perception of the patient's unconscious is more acute and active in advance of his conscious conception of the situation" (Langs, 1976, p. 78). Heimann, however, noted that pathological responses by the analyst could be used to understand the unconscious processes of the patient. The immediate emotional response of the analyst serves as a guide to the patient's unconscious processes and eventually a deeper understanding of the patient's personality (Heimann, 1950).

As Heimann noted, countertransference responses are a phenomenon caused by the patient and provide a window into the patient's unconscious. However, countertransference is a delicate matter that should be handled with caution, especially when the analyst has not gone through personal analysis. By going through personal analysis, the analyst is increasingly able to accept and handle the patient's projections when the patient reenacts their conflict within the therapeutic relationship. The lack of analysis can lead to analysts projecting their own unresolved issues onto the patient (Heimann, 1950). Heimann agreed with Freud's emphasis on analysts' need to "recognize and master" their own countertransference and emotional response to their patients; however, she rejected the need to detach as Freud suggested and considered this an extreme view. Instead, analysts should use their emotional responses to gain a greater insight into their patients' unconscious. Heimann also discouraged the sharing of countertransference responses with patients, as others before suggested, instead using the analyst's emotional responses for interpretation purposes only. Sharing the analyst's emotional response is counterproductive to treatment and places a burden on the patient. Emotions activated within the analyst are of value to treatment when used to gain insight into the patient's unconscious conflicts and defenses. When countertransference emotions are interpreted and worked on, changes within the patient's ego will occur, including the strengthening of the patient's reality sense, allowing them to see the analyst as simply another human being and not an object of idealization.

Margaret Little

Margaret Little expanded on the views of countertransference by exploring the interaction between the analyst's countertransference and the patient's response to it (Langs, 1976). According to Little (1981), most literature of the time focused on the transference dynamic of treatment; however, she emphasized that the basic tenets of transference were also relevant to that of countertransference. As a result, Little's (1981) definition of countertransference consisted of one or all four of the following possibilities:

1. The analyst's unconscious attitude toward the patient.
2. Repressed elements, hitherto unanalyzed, in the analyst himself which attach to the patient in the same way as the patient "transfers" to the analyst affects, etc., belonging to his parents or to objects of his childhood, that is, the analyst regards the patient (temporarily and varyingly) as he regards his own parents.
3. Some specific attitude or mechanism with which the analyst needs the patient's transference.
4. The whole of the analyst's attitudes and behaviors toward the patient. This includes all the others and any conscious attitude as well. (pp. 34–35)

Little finally settled on the definition of countertransference by using the symbol "R" as its representative. Little ultimately felt countertransference was best defined as "the analyst's total response to his patient's needs, whatever the needs, and whatever the response" (Little, 1981, p. 52). This view of countertransference covers all possible responses by the analyst, conscious and unconscious, and includes what they say, do, imagine, and feel toward the patient throughout the course of treatment (Little, 1981).

Along with the fact that psychological writings of the time were focusing on the transference phenomena, Little (1981) felt the lack of literature related to countertransference could also be attributed to the following:

1) Unconscious countertransference is something which cannot be observed directly as such, but only in its effects.
2) From a metapsychological standpoint, the analyst's total attitude involves his whole psyche, id, and any superego remnants as well as ego (he is also concerned with all these in the patient), and there are no clear boundaries differentiating them.
3) Any analysis (even self-analysis) postulates both the analysand and an analyst: in a sense they are inseparable. And similarly, transference and

countertransference are inseparable, something suggested in the fact that what is written about one can so largely be applied to the other.

4) The attitude toward countertransference, that is, toward one's own feelings and ideas, triggered a paranoid and phobic response by the profession as a result of having to identify, discuss and interpret feelings that were or may be subjective in nature. (p. 35)

In addition, the popular opinion at the time recognized the phenomenon of countertransference, however, considered it unnecessary and dangerous to interpret, similar to the resistance toward the use of transference within treatment in years prior (Little, 1981). Other issues revolved around the oversimplification in attempting to separate consciousness from the unconscious and ignoring the dynamics of the therapeutic relationship.

Little warned against the second form of countertransference and described it as the cause of "difficulties" and "dangers" related to treatment resulting from the pathological elements of the analyst's conscious and unconscious (Little, 1981). This, however, does not eliminate the element of the patient as the therapeutic relationship includes both transference and countertransference reactions that will always have a degree of closeness to both the patient and the analyst. Pathological elements, specifically repressed countertransference reactions, are creations of the unconscious part of the ego via the id, and are comparable to that of symptoms within patients. Like transference, countertransference reactions are concerned with another individual and will make themselves present through projections and introjections onto the patient. For instance, the analyst may unconsciously attempt to satisfy their libidinal needs by not only making incorrect interpretations but also ones that are necessary for the analyst, exploiting the patient's illness for the personal needs of the analyst. The patient becomes the analyst's "love object," whom they hope to make well while simultaneously making them dependent on the analyst by making them ill again. The repetitive cycle may lead to progress though if used correctly as the process will lead to the discovery of anxieties that could be interpreted and worked through. This in turn requires an unconscious willingness by the analyst to allow ego development on the part of the patient, leading to independence (Little, 1981). Incorrect or poorly timed interpretations play into the interdependence of the patient and analyst, eventually leading to the strengthening of the patient's resistance and re-repression.

When incorrect interpretations are made, Little encouraged the analyst to reveal their error while also exploring the countertransference resistance leading to the interpretation unless there is a contraindication in doing so. In such instances, the analyst should wait until the appropriate time to do so. The revelation promotes the growth of treatment, and it allows the patient to see the analyst as not only human but also as honest. Withholding such information would be counter indicative and harmful to the therapeutic relationship and treatment as a whole.

One key factor in the proper use of countertransference deals with the analyst's ability to distance and detach themselves from the patient's experience.

Unlike Freud, Little encouraged identifying and empathizing with the patient while still remaining distant. When an immediacy and presentness for the analyst with the patient's experience occurs, the analyst takes ownership of the experience as a result of the ego's inability to detach and distance themselves from the experience (Little, 1981). Proper ego functioning is necessary for the analyst to identify with the patient while also distancing themselves from the experience. According to Little (1981), "this detachment comes about partly at least by the use of the ego function of reality testing with the introduction of the factors of time and distance" (p. 39). When the analyst has gone through a similar experience to that of the patient, the detachment is created by the interval of time elapsed between the analyst and their experience, allowing for immediacy between the patient and the experience. The analyst knows it from the past while the patient knows it from their present situation, making it the patient's experience. If the experience is that of the patient alone, then an element of distance will be introduced automatically. Countertransference depends on the intervals of time and distance to be effective, a pastness resulting in the analyst's introjective identification with the patient. Time and distance within countertransference promote growth by prompting identification and separation for the patient (Little, 1981).

Little also addressed the use of countertransference when working with severely psychotic patients. According to Little (1981), when working with such populations, it is common for the analyst to identify with the patient's id as a result of the patient's shattered ego. Because of the disintegrated personality of the psychotic patient, the analyst's repressed material and primitive drives play a role in treatment, allowing for the patient's ego to identify with the unconscious part of the analyst's ego. Because the patient is unable to develop a transference for interpretation, the use of the analyst's countertransference is necessary to gain an understanding of the patient's inner world. Through the analyst's countertransference experience, the patient uses the analyst's libidinal energy and introjects the analyst's ego, providing an opportunity for them to come in contact with reality through the use of the analyst (Little, 1981). Through the free play of the analyst's unconscious impulses and fantasies, the analyst is able to overcome countertransference resistance and gain insight into the patient's unconscious (Langs, 1976). Little argued that such connection between the patient and analyst would lead to an intense emotional response and profound disturbance on the part of the analyst; however, this may be a reflection of the analyst identifying with the patient's id (Little, 1981).

Langs (1976) cautioned against the utilization of pathological countertransference responses. According to Langs (1976), "It is my impression that uncontrolled interventions based on countertransference difficulties, while they may evoke strong reactions in patients, in the main do not promote adaptive inner change" (p. 315). Langs (1976) added:

> There are many indications, however, that Little was quite aware of the dangers of such countertransference-based confrontations and that she

herself was uncertain regarding the management of these expressions in the relationship with the patient. Clearly those inner experiences that the analyst is able to recognize as derivatives of countertransference difficulties call for control and management on his part. He should not make interventions on such a basis until her has clarified the distortions in her perceptions of and reactions to the patient. He should then proceed with considerable caution, especially until her has engaged in a period of self-analysis in order to resolve as far as possible the basis for his countertransference difficulties.

(p. 315)

As Langs stated, Little does not encourage the unloading of countertransference interpretations without considering the negative effects on the client. However, she reminds us that countertransference responses are a result of the analytic work, a joint effort by the patient and analyst, and a reflection of the work as a whole. Little compares this to the analyst holding a mirror in front of the patient and the patient doing the same for the analyst, communicating through the mirroring of each other. As the analysis progresses, the mirror begins to lose its haze, providing clarity for the patient; however, as one mirror clears up, the same is expected of the other. The fog will remain if the countertransference is not explored (Little, 1981). Countertransference is not necessarily a pathological response by the analyst, but instead a projection belonging to the patient. Ignoring such a response would lead to the re-fogging of the mirror and a distancing from the analyst. The patient's uncertainty of the analyst will lead to the patient attempting to break down the analyst's resistances as a way of identifying with them and introjecting a part of the analyst and calling it their own, leading to a re-repression and greater resistance. Intense emotional responses should not be avoided and instead shared with the patient, allowing for the subjective understanding and recognition by both the patient and the analyst. If handled correctly, strong countertransference responses can provide an understanding of the patient's intrapsychic conflicts and unconscious fantasies (Langs, 1976).

According to Little (1981), one of the biggest emphases of treatment is placed on the unconscious fantasies of the patient onto their analyst; however, there also lies the resistance of the analyst. Through the course of treatment, patients come to learn a great deal about their analyst, yet they are unaware of such knowledge. It becomes the analyst's responsibility to bring such unconscious fantasies into consciousness. Disregarding the countertransference response is similar to ignoring its existence and making its knowledge and discussion of it taboo. Such stance prevents the patient's ego from understanding that the analyst has unconscious countertransference feelings toward them, hindering the accessibility of the patient's unconscious material.

Like those before her, Little also stressed the importance of the analysis of the analyst to remedy countertransference difficulties; however, she felt this was simply not enough, as it was impossible for analysts to become fully aware of their whole unconscious id, resulting in the development of unconscious infantile countertransference (Little, 1981). Although such countertransference is unavoidable, the aim through analysis is for a change in analysts' perspective toward their id impulses, no longer seeing them through a paranoid lens. A passive view related to the flooding of emotions toward one's patient leaves the analyst in a vulnerable state, resulting in the unconscious avoidance and denial of these emotions. The analyst's avoidance and insincerity will lead to the eventual hostility on the part of the patient. Open recognition of such emotions is an essential part of treatment and the therapeutic relationship, especially when the analyst services as a projection of the parental object. A resistance to that would lead to patients defending themselves through an introjection identification with the analyst instead of projecting the persecuting object onto the analyst. Recognizing and interpreting countertransference manifestations assist patients in understanding the development of their neurosis as a result of the parental figure's irrational behavior, allowing them to grow without interference or overstimulation. In other words, countertransference is not the greatest danger to treatment, but instead the greatest threat is posed by the views of the analyst toward countertransference (Little, 1981).

Complementary View – Heinrich Racker

Like the totalistic view of countertransference, the complementary view considered countertransference as an intricate part of treatment, seeing the analyst's internal response as inevitable, triggered by the patient's defenses and way of relating with others (Gelso & Hayes, 2007). The difference lies in the expression and communication between the conscious and unconscious processes within the patient and analyst. Within the therapeutic hour, the analyst and patient influence internal and external, conscious and unconscious responses within the other, resulting in a psychological dance, a push and pull of sorts between the two. According to Gelso and Hayes (2007), the patient will, both consciously and unconsciously, seek a certain response from the analyst, while the analyst will experience the need to respond to the patient's need, which in turn creates a response within the patient, resulting in a back and forth between the patient and the analyst. In other words, the analyst becomes the yin to the patient's yang, and vice versa, an interconnection between the two within the therapeutic relationship. Countertransference is then the psychic interaction between the patient and analyst and a complement to the patient's transference.

Heinrich Racker's writings on countertransference during the late 1950s continue to be influential within the field of psychoanalysis. Racker was critical of the lack of literature involving countertransference at the time and felt it was related to the psychoanalytic establishment simply denying their own countertransference. A rejection of countertransference was also a rejection of the analyst's primitive anxieties, guilt, and internal conflicts (Racker, 1988). Racker stated,

> [w]e must begin by revision of our feelings about our countertransference and try to overcome our own infantile ideals more thoroughly, accepting more fully the fact that we are still children and neurotics even when we are adults and analysts. Only in this way – by better overcoming our rejection of countertransference – can we achieve the same result in candidates.
> (p. 161)

Racker's view on countertransference expanded the perspectives set forth by Winnicott, Heimann, and Little, while also exploring the depths of the countertransference experience. Racker (1988) identified a number of guiding principles related to countertransference and emphasized the following:

> (1) Countertransference reactions of great intensity, even pathological ones, should also serve as tools; (2) Countertransference is the expression of the analyst's identification with the internal objects of the analysand, as well as with his id and ego, and may be used as such; and (3) Countertransference reactions have specific characteristics (specific content, anxieties, and mechanisms) from which we draw conclusions about the specific character of the psychological happenings in the patient.
> (p. 160)

In addition to seeing the beneficial use of countertransference, Racker brought to the forefront the psychic interaction between the analyst and patient, the push and pull within the transference/countertransference dynamic (Epstein & Feiner, 1988; Gordon et al., 2016). It is this push and pull between the analyst and patient that later played an intricate part in the development of the inter-subjective approach to countertransference.

According to Racker, countertransference served as a tool to understand the mental processes of patients, including their content, intensity, and manifestations; however, he also stressed the importance of analysts' awareness of their countertransference reaction, as acceptance allowed for an understanding of what material to interpret within treatment while also exploring the oedipal complex of the analyst toward the patient (Racker, 1968). Difficulties associated with countertransference result in difficulties with the analysis of the transference. Since the patient's transference involves the projection and expression of internal object relations, the analyst must have the capacity to relate to the patient's impulses, defenses, and internal objects, while simultaneously being aware of their identification. In other words, the analyst serves not only as the interpreter of the patient's unconscious processes but also as the object of such processes (Racker, 1968). The analyst's capacity to identify with the patient is determined by their willingness to accept their countertransference reaction since the analyst's countertransference is likely based on the identification with not only the patient's internal objects but also their own id and ego (Racker, 1968; Langs, 1976). If the analyst is unable to resolve their internal conflicts as a result of their own neurosis and unconscious inner world organization, then the analyst will encounter difficulties in the same manner as children do when they become adults, extending the mythology of the child within the mythology of the analytic situation. Instead of having the ability to analyze the patient's transference through the forms of projections related to the patient's object relations, the analyst will instead re-experience the events of their own childhood, influencing the analyst's behavior toward the patient as well as the process of treatment. Deficiencies in analyzing the patient's transference result from countertransference conflicts and the analyst's rejection of their countertransference response, preventing the analyst from identifying the patient's internal world. Analysis is not an interaction between a sick individual and a healthy one, but instead

> [a]n interaction between two personalities, in both of which the ego is under pressure from the id, the superego, and the external world, each personality has its internal and external dependencies, anxieties, and pathological defenses; each is also a child with its internal parents; and each of these whole personalities – that of the analysand and that of the analyst – respond to every event of the analytical situation.
>
> (Racker, 1988, p. 162)

Simply put, countertransference provides a conscious and unconscious mode of communication between the patient and analyst, however, in order for this communication and identification with the patient to take place, the analyst must have resolved their own internal conflicts.

Although such similarities exist between the personalities of the patient and analyst, Racker (1988) warned against the differences between the patient and analyst. One key difference is the analyst's position on objectivity, as the analyst's objectivity lies in their response to their subjectivity and countertransference reactions. True objectivity consists of the constant analysis and observation of the analyst's countertransference and subjectivity, ultimately leading to an objective stance with the patient. However, neurotic objectivity prevents the analysts from doing such, instead repressing their subjectivity and becoming submerged within their countertransference (Racker, 1988). Therefore, countertransference is the fusion between the past and present, a connection between fantasy and reality, internal and external, conscious and unconscious, depicting the totality of the psychological response of the analyst as a whole. Just as the patient's analytic experience consists of their transference predispositions and present reality, the analyst's analytic experience also consists of the same, resulting in their countertransference reaction (Racker, 1988).

According to Racker (1988), countertransference is analogous to transference. The patient's transference situation is the patient's complete psychological attitude of the analyst influenced by the patient's reality; however, they are experienced based on the patient's past and fantasies (Langs, 1976). Countertransference is therefore the totality of the analyst's psychological response, or the total countertransference experience (Langs, 1976). Racker (1988) classified countertransference into two different categories: direct and indirect countertransference. Direct countertransference is the result of a direct response to the patient, while indirect countertransference is a response related to an individual outside the therapeutic setting. Racker differentiates direct countertransference further and describes two different processes: concordant identification and complementary identification. Concordant identifications are centered on empathic responses by the analyst as they relate to the patient's thoughts and feelings and are based on introjection and projection. The analyst is able to feel and identify with the patient, and experience what the patient is feeling through their ability to empathize with them. The analyst begins to consciously experience what the patient is experiencing at an unconscious level, however unable to access (Corbett, 1987). Concordant identifications are an understanding of the patient's emotional state through the reproduction and re-experiencing of the analyst's past processes in response to the patient. According to Racker (1988),

> [w]e have the analyst as subject and the patient as object of knowledge, which in certain sense annuls the 'object relationship', properly speaking; and there arises in its stead the approximate union or identity between the subject's and the object's parts (experiences, impulses, defenses). The aggregate of the processes pertaining to that union might be designated, where necessary, 'concordant countertransference'.
>
> (p. 166)

In other words, concordant identifications are the analyst's identifications with the patient's id and/or ego (Racker, 1988; Epstein & Feiner, 1988).

On the other hand, complementary identifications are based on projections on the part of the patient as opposed to an identification with the patient's id or ego by the analyst. In the same fashion as the Kleinian concept of projective identification, complementary identifications serve as a primitive and self-preserving defense mechanism by the patient's ego involving two stages: the splitting and projection of the unwanted portion of the self. By splitting and projecting, patients are able to rid themselves of a toxic introject or an unwanted portion of the self or superego by identifying the unwanted portion of the personality within the analyst (Epstein & Feiner, 1988). They then begin to treat the analyst as an internal object, transforming the analyst into an object of persecution. As a result, the analyst's ego begins to identify with the patient's projections, leading to the analyst experiencing the projected feelings and impulses toward the patient (Racker, 1988; Epstein & Feiner, 1988). The negative transference response by the patient elicits a negative countertransference response by the analyst (i.e., the analyst is made to feel bad by the patient which in turn leads to the analyst seeing the patient as bad). Racker described this response as the *lex talionis*, the eye for an eye concept, a re-projection of the patient's projection, or the analyst's identification with the patient's persecuting internal objects. Because the law of talion reflects the ancient act of vengeance, the analyst seeks vengeance toward the patient as a result of the negative emotional response elicited by the patient. This, however, is limited to an identification not only with the patient's internal objects but also with a persecutory object, or internal object of the analyst, which is now being projected onto the patient (Racker, 1988; Epstein & Feiner, 1988). In other words, "we have an object relationship very like many others, a real 'transference' in which the analyst 'repeats' previous experiences, the patient representing internal objects of the analyst" (Racker, 1988, p. 166). As a result, the analyst feels threatened by their superego and internal objects, leading to the identification of the agent provocateur within the patient, or the analyst's object of persecution is projected onto the patient (Racker, 1988). If the analyst acts on anxieties brought on by their internal objects or a patient's projections, the patient is put in a situation where they re-experience and battle a reality based on their real and fantasized internal world, re-enforcing their beliefs of inadequacy and re-establishing the patient's neurosis (Langs, 1976). However, if the analyst is able to instead understand the importance of the situation at hand and identify with the patient's internal world through their own anxieties, the patient's ongoing cycle is interrupted, resulting in a positive countertransference experience (Racker, 1988).

Due to the interconnection between concordant and complementary countertransference, Racker encouraged the analyst's awareness of identifications with the patient in order to prevent a response related to the law of talion. If analysts reject a part of themselves (i.e., an aggressive part), they also reject a part of the patient, leading to a failed concordant identification and a greater complementary identification with the patient's rejecting object (Racker, 1988). The analyst's rejection also results in the analyst unifying with the patient's neurosis, and reinforcing the situation and perception that led to the patient's neurosis, hindering the progress of treatment. By accepting identification with the patient, the analyst becomes a container for the patient's feelings and impulses, allowing the analyst the opportunity to interpret their identification or countertransference response, linking the analyst's unconscious processes with that of the patient (Epstein & Feiner, 1988). Therefore, the analyst is able to understand what the projected object/imago invoked within them, using such experience as a way of interpreting the patient's transference. Once the patient becomes conscious of such projections and mechanisms, they become aware of their present reality not matching their internal perception, leading to an introjection based on reality as opposed to fantasy. This, however, only becomes possible if the analyst is conscious of their countertransference responses (Racker, 1988).

In addition to concordant and complementary countertransference responses, Racker divided the concept of countertransference even further. According to Racker (1988), countertransference responses are divided into countertransference thoughts and countertransference positions. A complementary countertransference would best describe a countertransference position. It is the analyst's emotional response brought on by the identification of the patient's internal objects or the analyst's object of persecution and/or internal objects. Countertransference thoughts, on the other hand, are identifications with the patient based on fantasy, spontaneous thoughts by the analyst linked to transference situations. It is the unification of the patient's and analyst's unconscious, or what Racker called the "psychological symbiosis" between two personalities (p. 172). The analyst's fantasy and reaction are based on their identification with themselves and the object toward which the desire is directed. The analyst is identifying with the patient's id, ego, or internal objects, and such identification serves as a potential source of information regarding the patient's inner world, and can assist in furthering the analysis. Through their thoughts, analysts may be able to identify what is repressed within the patient. However, for the analyst to identify with the patient, the potential for identification must be present. Racker (1988) added, "One may presume that every psychological constellation in the patient is brought into play in analysis. A symbiosis results, and now in the analyst spontaneously occur thoughts corresponding to the psychological constellation in the patient" (p. 172).

Racker (1988) identified a number of differences between countertransference thoughts and positions; however, the main difference is based on the degree to which the ego is involved with the experience. In one instance, the analyst's experience is based on thoughts and fantasy, with the experience having a low emotional intensity and response by the ego (i.e., countertransference thoughts). On the other hand, the analyst's countertransference experience involves a greater involvement of the ego and includes an intense emotional response by the analyst, leading to the perception of the experience being reality based and placing the analyst in a situation where they could be overtaken by their emotional response (i.e., countertransference position). In addition to the analyst's ego response to the experience, countertransference positions and responses also differ as a result of their origin. According to Racker (1988),

> The reaction experienced by the analyst as thought or fantasy arises from the existence of an analogous situation in the analysand – that is, from his readiness in perceiving and communicating his inner situation – whereas the reaction experienced with great intensity, even as reality, by the analyst arises from acting out by the analysand.
>
> (p. 173)

Racker (1988), however, does not dismiss the role the analyst plays within the experience. Racker added,

> [u]ndoubtedly there is also in the analyst himself a factor that helps determine the difference. The analyst has, it seems, two ways of responding. He may respond to some situation by perceiving his reactions, while others he responds by acting out (alloplastically or autoplastically). Which type of response occurs in the analyst depends partly on his own neurosis, on

his inclination to anxiety, on his defense mechanisms, and especially on his tendencies to repeat (act out) instead of making conscious. Here we encounter a factor that determines the dynamics of countertransference.

(p. 173)

In other words, the analyst can attempt to change their external environment based on the difficult situation encountered (alloplastic adaption), or attempt to change themself and their internal world and perceptions (autoplastic adaption). The intensity of the analyst's countertransference experience therefore becomes a defense and a resistance toward the remembrance and reenactment of early childhood experiences and internal conflicts (Racker, 1988). Racker warned against negative countertransference responses or a countertransference neurosis, a neurotic response brought on by the analyst's unresolved issues and internal conflicts. Although such responses are inevitable and brought on by the analyst's pathology, they still serve as a potential aid to the therapeutic relationship. Given that such responses are brought on by the patient's transference neurosis, the countertransference response could serve as a bridge in linking the internal word of the analyst to that of the patient, illuminating the patient's unconscious processes and aiding in understanding the patient's underlying issues and internal state (Gelso & Hayes, 2007). However, a negative countertransference response may trigger the analyst's neurosis, leading to the repression of the countertransference experience as a result of the analyst's ego or superego. Denying such aspects of the repression and/or experience denies the analyst a guide to understanding the patient's transference and internal world. As a result of the patient's transference toward the analyst, the patient will attempt to compensate for their perceived ego inferiority brought on by their internal objects. The patient will seek an equality with their internal objects through the use of the analyst "for in the patient's behavior there is an aggressiveness against these internal objects which the patient once experienced as superior and rejecting" (Racker, 1988, p. 178). Instead of repressing their countertransference reaction as a result of their narcissistic wound brought on by the patient's identification with their internal objects, the analyst should serve the same function as the patient's superego and make them conscious of their countertransference experience as such experience is also a response brought on by the analyst's identification with the patient's internal objects (Racker, 1988). To repress a countertransference response is to reject the identification with the patient's internal object, resulting in the patient re-experiencing the object of persecution. According to Racker (1988),

[i]f the analyst does not repress his deeper reactions to the analysand's associations and behavior, they will afford him an excellent guide for showing the patient these same repressed objects of his and the relationship in which he stands towards them.

(p. 178)

It is in this manner that it becomes possible to interrupt the patient's neurosis and cycle of re-living their previous experience, as countertransference responses are a direct reaction to the transference situation currently being experienced by the patient. An emotional response by the analyst, in particular frustration, depicts the exposure and interaction with the patient's bad object (Racker, 1988). By using the analyst's countertransference experience as a way to interpret the patient's internal world, the patient begins to experience and develop a different imago of the object currently present within the transference experience, with the patient introjecting a reality dissimilar to their internal perceptions (Langs, 1976).

According to Racker (1988), countertransference plays a vital role in obtaining a greater understanding of the patient's inner world; however, he warned of the possibility of seeing it as the "oracle" of treatment or a source of pure truth. Countertransference can provide great insight into the patient's psyche, but this would also require insight into the analyst's own internal processes. Racker stated:

> I think it certainly a mistake to find in countertransference reactions an oracle, with blind faith to expect of them the pure truth about the psychological situations of the analysand. It is plain that our unconscious is a very personal "receiver" and "transmitter" and we must reckon with the frequent distortions of objective reality. But it is also true that our unconscious is nevertheless "the best have of its kind." His own analysis and some analytic experience enables the analyst, as a rule, to be conscious of this personal factor and know his "personal equation."
>
> (p. 197)

Although Racker encouraged the need for personal therapy for analysts themselves, he still encouraged the use of countertransference as "the danger of exaggerated faith in the message of one's own unconscious is, even when they refer to very 'personal' reactions, less than the danger of repressing them and denying them any objective value" (p. 197). The analyst's emotional response, regardless of its possible neurotic origin, is a result of the patient's internal process and a response to the patient's transference. As a result, countertransference provides a view into the patient's psyche and their current situation, while providing a basis for interpretations and interventions (Langs, 1976).

Relational View – Lewis Aron

According to Aron (1993), the transference/countertransference dynamic within analysis is heavily influenced by the relationship and interactions between the patient and analyst. Unlike the classical view that considered much of the therapeutic process a result of the patient's pathology, the relational view emphasizes the co-construction of events within the therapeutic process, seeing the approach of analysis as a two-person psychology (Aron, 1993; Gelso & Hayes, 2007). As opposed to other conceptualizations of countertransference and psychodynamic theory that speak of the subjective experience and psychological independence within psychotherapy in comparison to the interplay between the patient and analyst such as the myth of the isolated mind (Stolorow & Atwood, 1996), the relational view does not anticipate an expected set of reactions on behalf of the analyst to the patient's covert and overt material. Instead, there is a mutual influence, a communication back and forth between the patient and analyst that determines the content of the transference and countertransference, shaping the nature of the transference/countertransference dynamic. Although the level of influence is not equal within the therapeutic relationship, there remains a continued mutual influence between the two. Countertransference is then a construct between the "inevitable interaction of the patient's dynamics (his or her transference, realistic expression, personality, etc.) and the therapist's dynamics (unresolved conflicts, personality, needs, realistic expression, etc.)" (Gelso & Hayes, 2007, p. 12).

The more traditional psychoanalytic approach and perception of treatment consist of the neurotic patient bringing their conflicts and defenses into treatment in order for them to be analyzed by the neutral, stable, objective, and well-analyzed analyst without taking the analyst's emotional experience into account as countertransference would signal the analyst's neurosis. On the other hand, other approaches consider all emotional responses by the analyst toward the patient as a source of countertransference, but not necessarily the analyst's pathology (Aron, 1991). This, however, exonerates the analyst of any responsibility for their countertransference response, as it is a direct response to the patient, making the analyst's experience reactive rather than subjective. As a result, the term countertransference "obscures the recognition that the analyst is often the initiator of the interactional sequence, and therefore the term minimizes the impact of the analyst's behavior on the transference" (Aron, 1991, p. 248). Instead, Aron (1991) argues that psychotherapy is an ongoing intrapsychic, influential, and circular interaction between the patient and analyst, and not a one-way psychological interaction. Aron (1996) stressed the importance of understanding the patient and analyst's ability to mutually regulate each other's state of consciousness in an "attempt to move regression out of the individual's mind and into the space between the participants. Thus we speak of mutual regression or of mutual regulation of regression" (p. 145).

According to Aron (1993), one of the key aspects of countertransference involves the patient's perception of the analyst. Due to the relational approach and ongoing cycle of mutual influence within the therapeutic relationship, it is important for the analyst to explore the patient's intersubjective experience with the analyst (Aron, 1993; Gelso & Hayes, 2007). According to Aron (1993), patients commonly tune in to the analyst's feelings and perceptions of them, both consciously and unconsciously. As a result of the ongoing communication between the patient and analyst, the patient is able to have an intersubjective experience with the analyst in the same fashion as the analyst has with the patient. Similar to the relationship between an infant and their mother, a patient, as a result of their unconscious phantasy, will seek to climb into and explore the analyst's internal world and the objects contained within. The patient is able to gather an understanding of the internal objects of the analyst and the relationship between them. But most importantly, the patient is able to formulate interpretations of the analyst's feelings and attitudes toward them. It becomes the patient's state of mind seeking the analyst's state of mind, allowing for the patient's psychic reality to bring the analyst's unconscious into consciousness (Aron, 1993). Patients, however, tend to discuss these observations of the analyst in an indirect manner, such as through displacements, allusions toward others, or identifications. Through the patient's intersubjective experience of the analyst, the analyst's countertransference becomes present within the therapeutic arena (Aron, 1993). According to Aron (1991), "An important aspect of making the unconscious conscious is to bring into awareness and articulate the patient's denied observations, repressed fantasies, and unformulated experiences of the analyst" (p. 251). These are simply not distortions or part of the patient's neurosis, but instead a possible reflection of the analyst's internal world needing to be explored within analysis. Therefore, a successful analysis using the two-person approach allows for the patient to understand their own psychology as well as the psychology of others through the patient's experience of the analyst's subjectivity (Wolstein, 1988; Aron, 1996).

Another aspect of the relational view on countertransference focuses on the analyst's bodily sensations, or somatic countertransference response to the patient (Aron, 1998). According to Aron (1998), the bodily experience of the analyst plays a central role within psychotherapy, as a result of the interconnectedness between the clinical body and the reflective mind, requiring the analyst "to move back and forth, and to maintain the tension, between a view of the self as a subject and a view of the self as an object" in what is known as self-reflexivity (p. 5). Through self-reflexivity, or the capacity to view oneself in both a subjective and objective manner, the analyst is able to access their bodily self, an experience that only becomes possible through the analyst's intersubjective experience. As a result of the interplay between the body–mind, mind–body phenomenon, the relational view on countertransference is not only a two-person psychology but also a two-body psychology.

As a way of distinguishing between subjective and objective awareness, Aron (1998) focuses on an individual's state of consciousness. For instance, with subjective awareness or subjective states of consciousness, individuals are completely immersed in their own thoughts and actions, and view themselves as the subject of their thoughts and actions. In contrast, with objective awareness or objective states of consciousness, the individual views themselves as the object of their thoughts and actions. As a result, Bach (1985) argued that an analyst is required to have the capacity to move from one state of consciousness to another, "both a subjectification and an objectification, two different perspectives on the same self" (p. 53). Ogden (1997) described the process of going between both states of consciousness in the following manner:

> Self-reflective thought occurs when "I" (as subject) look at "me" (as object). Metaphor is a form of language in which I describe "me" so that "I" might see myself. In an important sense, naming and describing "me" metaphorically creates both "I" and "me" as interdependent aspects of human self-awareness (human subjectivity). In other words, the individual (as object) is invisible to the self (as subject) until metaphors for "I" are used to describe or create "me" so that "I" can see myself. This is the mutually creating dialectic of "I" and "me."
>
> (p. 727)

If the analyst encounters difficulties moving between both states of consciousness, their ability to integrate both aspects of the self into their perception of the world becomes compromised. Trauma, according to Kalsched (1996), is one factor that has the ability to compromise and disrupt the analyst's capabilities of accessing both levels of consciousness, ultimately disrupting the mind–body connection.

According to Kalsched (2013), every patient has a story to tell and treatment does not begin until that story is told; however, he also mentioned that an individual is "often given more to experience in this life than we can bear to experience consciously" (p. 10). As a result, Kalsched argues that the psyche will depend on the sophisticated defenses of the unconscious to ensure survival and prevent the complete annihilation of the self resulting from trauma. To ensure its survival, the psyche will access what Kalsched (2013) calls the self-care system. However, under such circumstances, individuals are robbed of their opportunity to metabolize the trauma as they will dissociate and detach from the experience and distribute the unbearable affect to different parts of the psyche (Kalsched, 2013). As Kalsched (1996) stated:

> Because somatic and mental elements are "different," we might say that the self-care defense exploits the incommensurability between the mind and the body and divides up experience accordingly. The affect and sensation aspects of experience stay with the body and the mental representation aspect is split off into the "mind." Such a person will not be able to let somatic sensations and excited bodily states into mental awareness, i.e., will not be able to let his or her mind give shape to bodily impulses in words or images. Instead, messages from the body will have to be discharged in some other way and will therefore remain pre-symbolic. Such an individual will have no words for feelings, and this will put him or her at a terrible disadvantage.
>
> (p. 66)

In other words, the mind–body connection is severed, and the mind loses its ability to interpret the input received from the body and its senses. The different parts of the psyche cease to know each other, preventing the individual from experiencing the horrors of the trauma as a whole. As Kalsched (2013) stated, "Affect is split from image, body from mind, innocence from experience," as the psyche shatters, creating gaps within the experience while also separating the affect from the trauma and removing it from consciousness (p. 89). The splitting of the psyche preserves the aliveness of the individual and preserves the traumatic memories within the unconscious in order for the person to digest them when they are psychologically ready to do so. Through dissociation, the individual preserves a vital core of the self by removing it from the experience and the suffering of reality. In a way, the person becomes the reflection of Lucifer, the fallen angel that separated himself from the heavens as a result of being unable to tolerate God's plan (Kalsched, 2013).

As a way of re-establishing the mind–body connection, Kalsched (2013) argues the importance of the analyst learning the language of the soul as it is the human soul that is threatened with annihilation as a result of the trauma. In learning the language, treatment becomes more effective, since the traumatic experience is provided with an opportunity and a voice to be heard, allowing for the restoration and integration of the shattered psyche. Such language is visible through psychic openings that consist of flashbacks, dreams, and the transference. By integrating the language of the soul, the integration of the psyche and the individualization of the self becomes possible, providing the individual with an arena for tolerating and metabolizing the suffering in order for it to become a memory (Kalsched, 2013). The analyst therefore re-establishes the severed connection between the mind and body.

Integrative View – Charles Gelso and Jeffery Hayes

Through their research and clinical experience spanning over two decades, Gelso and Hayes (2007) have developed a conception of countertransference that looks at all four of the previously discussed views and integrated certain aspects of each. According to Gelso and Hayes (2007), countertransference is defined as "the therapist's internal or external reactions that are shaped by the therapist's past or present emotional conflict and vulnerabilities" (p. 25). Although Gelso and Hayes argued that countertransference was a co-creation of the analyst and patient within the therapeutic relationship, the analyst's emotional conflicts and vulnerabilities must be involved and affected in order for the response to be considered countertransference (Gelso & Hayes, 2007). In addition, the emotional conflicts and vulnerabilities reflect the analyst's past in the form of past experiences, including childhood experiences, now locked in the analyst's unconscious. For the most part, the analyst's experiences remain latent and are rarely activated within their everyday lives; however, the therapeutic area poses a different threat for the analyst as memories may be stimulated by some aspect of the patient. In both cases, the analyst's reaction is triggered by the patient's behavior or relatable experience. In such situations where the analyst's conflicts are activated, the analyst's reactions are similar to the transference response by the patient with the patient representing a key figure of the analyst's past or present (Gelso & Hayes, 2007).

In addition to the conflicts and vulnerabilities of the analyst, Gelso and Hayes (2007) also stress the importance of the internal and external responses of the analyst. Internal reactions consist of thoughts, feelings, emotions, and body sensations experienced by the analyst. On the other hand, external responses consist of verbal and nonverbal responses or behaviors the analyst exhibits toward the patient (Gelso & Hayes, 2007). When using countertransference as a tool within treatment, it is important for the analyst to be aware of what is going on internally, whether in the form of thoughts or feelings, within the therapeutic hour as well as outside of it. Ideally, the analyst should attempt to understand what is happening within their psyche as opposed to simply looking at what the patient is doing to create such responses. Only by being aware of such responses does it become possible for the analyst to achieve empathic understanding of the patient, in addition to being responsive to the feelings being expressed by the patient. According to Gelso and Hayes (2007), "The road to understanding likely begins with a sense in the therapist that something is awry emotionally" during the therapeutic hour (p. 28). Such awareness can also take place outside of the therapeutic hour and should serve as a cue that something internally is not quite right for the analyst. At a minimum, the analyst should become more observant of their actions in order to determine the cause of their response.

Internal countertransference responses by the analyst are inevitable within treatment. Generally speaking, internal countertransference is the result of the development of unresolved issues and vulnerabilities throughout the analyst's life. Although therapy plays a critical role in the analyst's ability to overcome such conflicts and vulnerabilities, the analyst does not simply solve such difficulties but instead learns to deal with them. As a result, the analyst will always be vulnerable to the patient's material. This, however, allows for an empathic connection with the patient, assuming that the analyst is able to manage and understand the source of their own response. When the conflicts and vulnerabilities being triggered are not too great in intensity, it is possible that the analyst is experiencing a similar reaction to those stimulated by the patient in other individuals (Gelso & Hayes, 2007). Such a response by the analyst provides the analyst with a glimpse of how the patient affects others. Ultimately, it is important to understand that countertransference is a result of the patient's underlying needs, wishes, and fears; hence, understanding one's countertransference provides an understanding of the patient's needs, wishes, and fears within the therapeutic relationship as well as the patient's relationship with others (Gelso & Hayes, 2007).

When looking at external countertransference reactions, Gelso and Hayes (2007) are referring to the countertransference manifestations seen in the analyst's behavior toward the patient. Such manifestations present themselves in a number of ways and can be seen in subtle ways. External countertransference responses represent the acting out of the analyst's internal countertransference response. Due to the analyst's blind spots in their internal responses, the analyst becomes aware of their countertransference as a result of acting out. In certain circumstances, the acting out on the part of the analyst is a way of keeping their internal countertransference unconscious, a way of preventing the analyst from dealing with a painful or uncomfortable situation, making it necessary for the analyst to monitor their response toward the patient (Gelso & Hayes, 2007).

Clinical Case Example – The Heroine in Disguise

HR began working with Scarlett after Scarlett requested a change in her mental health provider. Scarlett was a queer woman in her late thirties and was receiving treatment from a local community-based mental health program. Scarlett had a diagnosis of borderline personality disorder and engaged in severe and persistent self-harm and suicidal behaviors, including 40 prior suicide attempts. Scarlett had a history of overwhelming her therapists, including driving a prior therapist into their own suicidal crisis. During their first session, HR felt an immense pressure to get Scarlett to buy into treatment and felt as if "I only had one shot at getting it right, a pressure to say all of the right things." Once HR and Scarlett were able to develop a strong therapeutic bond that allowed them to work on core issues, HR found herself having rescue fantasies about rescuing Scarlett.

HR's rescue fantasies consisted of thinking "it would never happen" if she could not facilitate healing for Scarlett. HR found herself thinking that if she cared for Scarlett enough, if she were a good-enough therapist, then Scarlett would not kill herself. This belief was strengthened by Scarlett's comment that HR was her only reason to live. In addition, Scarlett attempted to negotiate with HR by promising not to self-harm in exchange for longer sessions or check-ins throughout the week. The initial pressure to get buy-in had now turned into pressure to "get it right" so Scarlett would choose to live. HR realized that she was putting full responsibility onto herself for Scarlett's choice to live or die, although she knew intellectually that was not the case. Despite being fully aware of this, HR continued having fantasies that only she could save Scarlett, and that no other therapist was capable of facilitating healing.

As a way of metabolizing her countertransference reaction, HR allowed herself to sit with her feelings and reactions in an attempt to understand them better. She was intentional in not feeling a sense of shame about them and instead used them as a source of information to gain a deeper understanding of Scarlett while also determining how to proceed with treatment. In further analyzing her response, HR realized that Scarlett was likely eliciting these reactions partly because of her extensive trauma history, which included abuse and abandonment by her caregivers. Rather than attempting to rescue her, HR shifted and instead focused on providing Scarlett with a corrective emotional experience through the processing of her trauma. It also allowed Scarlett to experience healing resulting from her effort and dedication to treatment, thus empowering her while counteracting HR's rescue fantasies. HR was now working with Scarlett as opposed to working for her.

The countertransference experience provided HR with the understanding of Scarlett's relational pattern of becoming extremely close to someone until she became "too much" for them, resulting in the reoccurring theme of abandonment. HR experienced the same pull to help Scarlett as others; however, she was able to identify it before it "drained" her. HR's countertransference experience also assisted in understanding the depth of Scarlett's pain, allowing her to become more attuned to her chronic sense of hopelessness. This attunement helped Scarlett reduce her shame about suicidality, allowing her to process it fully and develop a sense of hope and identify reasons to live.

HR's countertransference response ultimately allowed for a more authentic therapeutic relationship and a more accurate understanding of Scarlett. Therapy sessions began flowing smoothly as HR no longer felt the pressure to "get it right" and instead entrusted Scarlett to have vulnerable conversations that would facilitate healing. In addition, Scarlett developed trust toward HR while also sensing her self-assuredness that things were moving in the right direction, and that things "would get better." At the time of termination, Scarlett was no longer self-harming or engaging in suicidal behaviors. She felt safer in her body, was experiencing fewer symptoms, and became future-oriented.

3 Countertransference and Jungian Analysis

One of the main focal points of Jungian analysis is the use of countertransference, or the experience of the analyst. Like Freud, Carl Jung based his methodology on the analysis of transference. It is the push and pull of the transference/countertransference dynamic between the patient and analyst that speaks volumes even in silence.

> For all projections provoke counter-projections when the object is unconscious of the quality projected by the subject, in the same way that a transference is answered by a counter-transference from the analyst when it projects a content of which he is unconscious but which nevertheless exists in him.
>
> (Jung, 1948/1969, p. 273)

However, defining countertransference from a Jungian perspective can be difficult, as there is no general consensus among analytical psychologists (Machtiger, 1982). The differing definitions are dependent on the view embraced by the analyst. The more traditional view defines and limits countertransference as "the unconscious projections or feelings incurred by the analyst in reaction to the attitudes and products of the patient" (Machtiger, 1982, p. 88). This approach does not account for a number of factors relevant to countertransference, such as the conscious and preconscious attitudes of the analyst, or the positive and negative reactions associated with the therapeutic relationship. Instead, countertransference brings forward the unconscious aspects of the analyst's psyche, making them the focal point of treatment.

The more contemporary view of countertransference favors a broader definition, considering all aspects of the therapeutic experience as countertransference manifestations. Unlike the more traditional views of countertransference, contemporary views use the analyst's conscious responses to the real or imagined perception of the patient as a way of gaining an understanding of the interpersonal relationship between the patient and analyst. The sum of these parts depicts the psychic reality of the analyst, a reality created through a dialectic process between two individuals (Jung, 1935/1970). Jung (1935/1970) wrote, "A person is a psychic system which, when it affects another person,

DOI: 10.4324/9781003320180-4

enters into a reciprocal reaction with another psychic system" (p. 3). Through this relationship, the psyche of the analyst and the patient interact between the realms of consciousness and the unconscious.

Although Freud (1910/1953) originally coined the term *countertransference*, Jung was the first to integrate its meaning within the framework of analysis (Machtiger, 1982). For Jung, analysts undergo constant stress during the analysis of patients, making them susceptible to countertransference. Like Freud, Jung was of the belief that analysts, like patients, have blind spots and complexes that could interfere with the progress of treatment. Jung saw countertransference as an "occupational hazard" and warned of a potential "psychic infection" (Jung, 1937/1970; Jung, 1958/1969). Jung (1937/1970) warned:

> Even if the analyst has no neurosis, but only a rather more extensive area of unconsciousness than usual, this is sufficient to produce a sphere of mutual unconsciousness, i.e., a counter-transference. This phenomenon is one of the chief occupational hazards of psychotherapy. It causes psychic infections in both analyst and patient and brings the therapeutic process to a standstill.
>
> (pp. 329–330)

In addition, Jung equated countertransference to the demon of sickness, stating, "a sufferer can transmit his disease to a healthy person whose powers then subdue the demon – but not without impairing the well-being of the subduer" (Jung, 1931/1970, p. 72). As a result, Jung urged analysts to undergo their own personal analysis as a way of uncovering their own personal blind spots, as "the patient's treatment begins with the doctor, so to speak. Only if the doctor knows how to cope with himself and his own problems will he be able to teach the patient to do the same" (Jung, 1989, p. 132). Analysis requires the analyst to go through an infinite learning cycle. With each patient capable of uncovering the analyst's unconscious material previously in hibernation, the analyst is required to frequently learn about himself or herself (Jung, 1951/1970). Through analysis can the analyst learn to know his or her own psyche. If the analyst is unable to do so, treatment becomes stagnant and the patient is unable to learn as a result of the analyst not knowing how to cope himself or herself. The analyst, like the patient, will lose a portion of his or her psyche as it goes into the unconscious, making the analysis of the analyst the sine qua non of treatment (Jung, 1989). The analyst gains the ability to heal by understanding his or her own hurt. Wounds should not be feared but embraced, as "they can be the measure of one's healing power" (Merchant, 2012, p. 6). Through a connection with psychological wounds, the analyst develops a greater sense of empathy, as "the doctor is effective only when he himself is affected. Only the wounded physician heals" (Jung, 1989, p. 134). This again stresses the importance of analysts knowing themselves, by way of their own analysis, as a way of assisting their patients with gaining a greater understanding of themselves.

By understanding their personal wounds can the analyst understand the patient (Cvetovac & Adame, 2017).

Through a deeper understanding of themselves, analysts become capable of understanding their patients. In this view, countertransference is not a hindrance to treatment, but a vital component within analysis and a therapeutic instrument illuminating the patient's unconscious through the use of the analyst's psyche, straying away from Freud's view of it being an "unnecessary containment" (Machtiger, 1982). In Jungian psychology, countertransference experiences place analysts at the forefront of their own psyche, allowing them to use it as a valuable tool to understand their patients at a more profound level. In addition, Jungian analysis incorporates an archetypal dimension to the use of countertransference. The analyst's countertransference reactions provide an avenue to understanding the patient's archetypal influences and view of the archetype as a whole (i.e., savior/sinner), while simultaneously providing the analyst with information as to what is occurring during treatment (Kaufmann, 1984).

From a Jungian perspective, the unconscious also makes itself present in the form of *archetypes*. Jung broke down the unconscious into two distinct structures: the personal and collective unconscious. The personal unconscious is derived from the patient's personal experiences and consists mostly of an individual's complexes, with the material being conscious at one point or another. In contrast, the collective unconscious is not acquired but is inborn; it is not individualized but is universal (Jung, 1954/1969). Unlike the personal unconscious, the content of the collective unconscious has never been conscious, never acquired, and instead owes its existence to heredity (Jung, 1954/1969). Jung argued that the collective unconscious houses the

> [c]ontents and modes of behaviour that are more or less the same everywhere and in all individuals. It is, in other words, identical in all men and thus constitutes a common psychic substrate of a suprapersonal nature which is present in every one of us.
>
> (Jung, p. 4)

This content, what Jung called the "representations collectives" or the primitive perception of the world, is the archetypal material of the unconscious, a psychic representation yet to make itself conscious (Jung, 1954/1969). In addition to psychic representations associated with archetypal projections, the collective unconscious is also connected to the shadow, or the disowned part of an individual. Although Jung described the acknowledgment of the shadow as unpleasant to the conscious aspect, he viewed it as an intricate part of treatment and a necessary step toward healing and gaining a greater understanding of one's self.

Acknowledging the existence of one's *shadow* material is a necessity for healing, as it enables individuals to know themselves by bringing their personal unconscious to light and preparing for deeper exploration into the collective unconscious (Jung, 1954/1969). Jung described the process of venturing into the unconscious in the following fashion:

> The shadow is a tight passage, a narrow door, whose painful constriction no one is spared who goes down to the deep well. But one must learn to know oneself in order to know who one is. For what comes after that door is, surprisingly enough, a boundless expanse full of unprecedented uncertainty, with apparently no inside and no outside, no above and no below, no here and no there, no mine and no thine, no good and no bad. It is the world of water, where all life floats in suspension; where the realm of the sympathetic system, the soul of everything living, begins; where I am indivisibly this *and* that; where I experience the other in myself and the other-than-myself experiences me.
>
> (pp. 21–22)

The collective unconscious is not a personal system, but instead an endless world of possibilities, as "there are as many archetypes as there are typical situations in life" (Jung, p. 48). Archetypal representations are "forms without content," providing a number of possible perceptions and/or actions. In a situation relevant to an archetype, the archetype is activated and actualized through the experience of the individual (Adams, 2008). According to Jung (1918/1964), archetypes "do not produce any contents of themselves" but instead "give definite form to contents that have already been acquired" through experiences (pp. 10–11). The archetype alone is meaningless, shapeless, but through the constellating experience of the archetype we impose meaning and form on the content of the archetype. The archetype alone is a potential form of the unconscious, similar to the guiding principles of snowflake formation (Gieser, 2005; B. McDavitt, personal communication, November 26, 2015). The formation of snowflakes is a universal phenomenon following the same formula each time; however, each snowflake remains unique in its own right, influenced by a number of different factors during formation. Like snowflakes, archetypes are inborn and universal as well but still individualized from person to person based on the random vicissitudes and experiences of life. According to Gieser (2005),

> [t]he archetype must not be seen as "causing" the constellation, any more than the hexagonal structure of the snowflake "causes" the appearance of the individual snowflake. The archetype "in itself" has nothing at all to do with a visual or known structure; it is rather a "possibility of structure", which in addition contains an affective or qualitative element rather than an abstract geometrical one.
>
> (p. 290)

Archetypes and potential archetypal manifestations are therefore experience driven and dependent on the aspects of the experience that activate and place meaning on the archetype.

Archetypal manifestations present themselves in a number of different ways; however, due to their unconscious content, their conscious manifestation becomes an alteration of the unconscious, as they take their meaning from the individual experiencing the conscious material (Jung, 1954/1969). Within analysis, archetypal material is projected onto the patient or the analyst; however, the duality of the archetype is not projected as a whole (i.e., animus/anima, wise man/fool). Instead, the portion missing within the individual, giving the analyst the option of amplifying and returning the projection, or incarnating and becoming "what the patient's unconscious insists I should be" (Plaut, 1956, p. 157). However, archetypal projections also occur within the analyst, caused by the same lack of integration and identification of the archetype as a whole (i.e., difficulty with the embodiment of archetypal evil). If the analyst does not stay conscious of the duality of the archetype in some capacity, the unconscious portion will be projected onto the patient, transforming the patient into what the analyst's unconscious insists they should be.

According to Jacoby (1984), the analyst will embody the patient's archetypal projections in both positive and negative forms; however, the analyst's countertransference response is dependent on the archetypal element being projected and their identification with it. In the ideal situation, the analyst is able to embody the archetypal image projected by the patient without identifying with it, allowing the patient and analyst to experience the archetype as a whole (Plaut, 1956). However, if analysts identify with the archetypal projection, they are "rendered incapable of maintaining and sustaining that balance that facilitates the patient's disidentification from the archetypal image" (Machtiger, 1982, p. 97). As a result, Jung (1954/1969) warned that individuals

> who descends into the unconscious gets into a suffocating atmosphere of egocentric subjectivity, and in this blind alley is exposed to the attack of all the ferocious beasts which the caverns of the psychic underworld are supposed to harbour.
>
> (p. 20)

Unlike the process of analysis, in which the analyst helps the patient work through projections and unconscious material, the analyst examines his or her material independently, attempting to own and sort out personal projections. According to B. McDavitt (personal communication, November 26, 2015), the patient can play an instrumental role in assisting the analyst in uncovering and understanding his or her archetypal projections. In such instances, the patient will inform the analyst of distortions occurring in treatment or express concerns over the perceived confusion of the analyst, allowing for a shared experience between the patient and the analyst as a result of the psychic energy brought on by the therapeutic relationship. Archetypal aspects of countertransference originate through the shared unconscious relationship of the patient and analyst, a middle ground between fantasy and reality known as the *participation mystique* (Machtiger, 1982). Participation mystique is a representation of the psychological connections between patient and analyst, a shared oneness brought on by the therapeutic relationship that allows the individuals to identify with each other through a shared influence or experience (Jung, 1971). As a result, the transcendent function activates and provides an opportunity for healing and growth for those involved, furthering the process of individuation by creating transitions between attitudes, stages of development, and the usage of symbols (Machtiger, 1982). Through the use of symbols, it becomes viable to bridge archetypal opposites and unites opposite trends, leading to the eventual goal of wholeness.

Projections and introjections are important components of countertransference, as they are capable of influencing the therapeutic relationship by making unconscious material a conscious reality through an archetypal or metaphorical representation of the unconscious (Paulsen, 1956). Projections and introjections provide countertransference manifestations with their appearance, translating unconscious processes into conscious ones. Through introjections, the analyst can identify, empathize, or sympathize with the patient; however, hostile responses are also possible. These mental functions transform the analyst into an instrument that aids in the furthering of treatment. In addition, countertransference requires the analyst to accept and understand the patient's feelings of pain and states of confusion. By serving as a container for the patient, the potential for growth becomes possible, allowing the analyst to gain information through countertransference reactions in order to understand the patient's unconscious material (Paulsen, 1956). In addition, archetypal relationships are expressed through the alchemical process in the form of projections, providing a link between the past and present, and the psychology of the unconscious (Jung, 1968b). According to Jung,

[t]he method of alchemy, psychologically speaking, is one of boundless amplification. The *amplificatio* is always appropriate when dealing with some dark experience which is so vaguely adumbrated that it must be enlarged and expanded by being set in a psychological context in order to be understood at all.

(Jung, p. 289)

Amplification is therefore a necessity within analytical psychology, as it enriches the archetypal content through the amplification of symbols and experiences within treatment to the point where it is understood and experienced by both the analyst and the patient.

Countertransference is viewed as an activation of the analyst's unconscious brought on by the patient's transference projections, making it an inevitable phenomenon within psychotherapy. As a result, Jung viewed countertransference as an "inductive" phenomenon originating within the patient, but developing and growing within the analyst's unconscious (Newman, 1980). Meier (1959) explained, "It may be assumed that the 'catching' of projections by a 'hook' cannot be without effects on the carrier, and that a counter-effect will not be lacking" (p. 23). Countertransference is therefore a reciprocal unconscious relationship between the patient and the analyst, and a prerequisite to resolving the patient's transference (Sedgwick, 1994). Jung (1931/1970) explained,

> [f]or, twist and turn the matter as we may, the relationship between the doctor and patient remain a personal one within the impersonal framework of professional treatment. By no devise can the treatment be anything but the product of mutual influence, in which the whole being of the doctor as well as that of his patient plays its part. In the treatment there is an encounter between two irrational factors, that is to say, between two persons who are fixed and determinable quantities but who bring with them, besides their more or less clearly defined fields of consciousness, an indefinitely extended sphere of non-consciousness. Hence the personalities of doctor and patient are often infinitely more important for the outcome of treatment than what the doctor says and thinks (although what he says and thinks may be a disturbing or a healing factor not to be underestimated). For two personalities to meet is like mixing two different chemical substances: if there is any combination at all, both are transformed. In any effective psychological treatment the doctor is bound to influence the patient; but this influence can only take place if the patient has a reciprocal influence on the doctor.
>
> (p. 71)

Jung referred to countertransference as a symptom of the patient's transference; however, Jung was not referring to a reactive response on behalf of the analyst to the patient's transference. Instead, he was referring to the transfer of the patient's illness to the analyst through unconscious influences (Sedgwick, 1994). This led to Jung's criticism of Freudian techniques and theory in general, seeing them as counterproductive and as a way that analysts could shield themselves from the patient's influential illness. Jung understood the power of the patient's affect and effects it could have on the analyst. The analyst's introjections and responses to the patient's affect are what Jung considered countertransference.

As a way of describing the psychic interactions between the unconscious of the patient and analyst, Jung used the alchemical process, more specifically the *coniunctio*, or the divine marriage, as a metaphorical explanation. Through alchemy, the mystic marriage involves the unification of chemical substances in hopes of discovering a new substance, or as was the case for alchemists, the chemical combination that produced gold (Jung, 1946/1970). Alchemists observed and experimented with each chemical substance and noted their interactions as they became evident. The unconscious of the patient and analyst interact in the same fashion, describing the dance between the transference/countertransference dynamic that takes place in the therapeutic relationship. Through this interaction, Jung anticipated the psychological infection of the analyst and encouraged its acceptance as part of the therapeutic process.

According to Jung, the analyst "should clearly understand that psychic infections, however superfluous they seem to him, are in fact the predestined concomitants of his work" (Jung, 1946/1970, p. 177). Jung (1946/1970) added,

> [t]he doctor by voluntarily and consciously taking over the psychic suffering of the patient, exposes himself to the overpowering content of the unconscious and hence also to their inductive action. . . . The patient, by bringing an activated unconscious content to bear upon the doctor, constellates the corresponding unconscious material in him, owing to the inductive effect which always emanates from projections in greater or lesser degree. Doctor and patient thus find themselves in a relationship founded on mutual unconsciousness.
>
> (pp. 175–176)

Alchemically speaking, the unconscious of both the patient and the analyst begins their unification and transformation, the divine marriage leading to the creation of a third component, and in the case of the patient, toward the direction of healing. Through this premise, Jung reminds us that treatment is a dialectical process, a process in which the analyst's participation is just as important as that of the patient (Jung, 1951/1970). Jung (1931/1970) stated,

> [f]or two personalities to meet is like mixing two different chemical substances: if there is any combination at all, both are transformed. In any effective psychological treatment the doctor is bound to influence the patient; but this influence can only take place if the patient has a reciprocal influence on the doctor. You can exert no influence if you are not susceptible to influence.
>
> (p. 71)

Countertransference is more than simply a projection on behalf of the analyst, it is the interaction and lived experience between the patient and analyst. Through countertransference reactions, it becomes possible to gain an understanding of what is going on within analysis. In other words, the closer the analyst is to his or her countertransference response, the further the patient has traveled down the road of healing.

Clinical Case Example – The Trapped Inner Lion

Tom reached out to MK at his wife's suggestion. Tom sought treatment to address the ongoing conflict between him and his wife. MK described Tom as a quiet man in his mid-thirties. Tom presented as visibly frustrated during sessions; however, he was "a man of few words." Approximately, 2 months into treatment, MK experienced a sense of reverie while sitting in silence with Tom. As she returned her attention to Tom, she noticed that Tom was soothing himself by petting a fluffy accent pillow that suddenly appeared to take the shape of a lion and its mane. MK looked away on several occasions; however, the shape remained on the pillow for the remainder of the session. MK could not explain the phenomenon, especially since the same pillow did not take the shape of the lion with any other patient. However, once Tom returned the following week, the shape of the lion returned.

At this point, MK became aware that she had a countertransference experience through the use of her imagination. MK felt the image was made possible by the transcendent function and the interaction between the unconscious of Tom and MK. MK initially considered the image to represent treatment and the therapeutic relationship and began contemplating Tom's effect on her. MK felt confused by the image and felt it contradicted Tom's demeanor. Although MK felt confused by the image, she believed it offered some insight into Tom's psyche and continued to metabolize the image internally.

As MK continued to examine her countertransference experience, she returned to the therapeutic relationship and Tom's hesitation to express himself. Tom appeared stuck and expressed his anger through silence. Before seeing the image of the lion, there was a long moment of silence between Tom and MK and a foggy sense of confusion. In Tom's silence, there was a constant rage that remained unspoken as Tom learned early on in his marriage that showing any signs of anger or aggression was considered unacceptable. In addition, Tom was expected to focus on his family and, as a result, distanced himself from his friends and stopped playing baseball, one of his favorite activities to release stress and frustration. In treatment, MK and Tom were stuck, and there was nothing more than the constant reenactment of anger through silence, preventing treatment from progressing. As the analyst, MK was experiencing a form of projective identification in that she was paralyzed just like Tom and not knowing in what direction to take in treatment.

As a way of further digesting the image of the lion, MK began to engage in an active imagination to see what information could be used to amplify Tom's feeling stuck. In MK's imagination, she saw the lion and perceived it as a wild and untamable creature, a creature that is safe at a distance and when left alone with its pride, yet dangerous if approached or if it perceives you as a threat. Through her internal dialogue, MK began to see a conscious image of what was previously unconscious, a lion who felt threatened after being separated from its pride and having to wander the Earth on its own. Tom was that lonely lion who required ongoing soothing to deal with the loneliness. Although MK did not disclose the image of the lion to Tom, she did share with him the understanding the image evoked in her, allowing treatment to progress.

Through the use of active imagination, MK was able to detach herself from the fused unconscious state she shared with Tom, bringing the stuck transference into consciousness. The image from Tom's unconscious manifested in the transcendent function, allowing MK to transform the image through her internal workings while also bringing it into consciousness via symbolic interpretation.

4   Countertransference Dreams

The concept of countertransference dreams has gone through a similar evolution as that of countertransference; however, the available literature on the
subject remains scarce. According to Zwiebel (1985), the lack of countertransference dream material is related to a number of factors including the change in
prominence and significance of dreams within analytic treatment, the negative
perception of countertransference dreams that views the phenomenon as a disturbance within the analyst and as a disturbance to treatment, and the analyst's
difficulty differentiating between the manifest and latent content of the dream.
In addition, countertransference dreams pose a threat of exposure to analysts
related to their own neurosis (Pollack-Gomolin, 2002). Early writings on the
subject implemented a classical view that focused on the analyst's neurosis,
whereas later writings focus on the analyst's full experience of the patient, or
the analyst's intersubjective experience of the patient. As a way of deciphering
the different views on countertransference dreams, psychoanalytic literature
categorizes countertransference dreams into three distinct categories: neurotic
countertransference dreams, projective identification dreams, and intersubjective dreams.

Neurotic Countertransference Dreams

Neurotic countertransference dreams look at dreams through the classical lens
of countertransference, meaning that the origin of such dreams is located within
the analyst's unconscious and is related to the analyst's neurosis. In more specific terms, neurotic countertransference dreams consist of dreams associated
with the analyst's anxiety related to working with a patient or patients. Given
that neurotic countertransference dreams tend to take place during difficult
phases of treatment, common themes associated with such dreams include the
analyst's level or loss of competence (Tauber, 1988; Jung, 1968b; Zwiebel,
1985), links between the analytic situation and the analyst's past experiences
and/or complexes, disturbances within the analytic relationship (Zwiebel,
1985), the analyst's neurotic distortions (Abramovitch & Lange, 1994), and
the analyst's acting out (Gitelson, 1952). According to Zwiebel (1985), most
countertransference dreams, in particular, neurotic countertransference dreams,

DOI: 10.4324/9781003320180-5

originate from a feared loss of competence within the analyst. Neurotic counter-transference dreams tend to be intense in nature and commonly share a link to the analyst's personality and/or internal conflicts. The analyst's perceived loss of competence can result in difficulties in understanding and being understood, feelings of hopelessness, and the reigniting of memories of the analyst's past experiences and/or trauma. Analysts commonly attempt to avoid the remembrance of such experiences, especially if they have not had the opportunity to work through them. However, neurotic countertransference dreams expose analysts to their repressed memories while also providing an opportunity for a reparative experience. In other words, if analysts use the dream to work through their neurosis, the countertransference dreams can eventually lead to the reinstatement of the analysts' competence that was previously disrupted.

The first documented countertransference dream is Freud's (1910/1953) dream commonly known as "Irma's injection." Freud's dream was about his former patient Irma after being informed by his colleague, Otto, that she was not doing well. This news led Freud to complete a case history on Irma's treatment the night before the dream. In the dream, Freud found himself hosting a social gathering, with Irma being one of the guests in attendance. As Freud notices Irma, he pulls her aside to reproach her for not accepting his treatment recommendations. Irma responded by informing Freud of her worsening medical condition. Irma's comments, in addition to her appearance, led to Freud's immediate examination of Irma. His examination led to the discovery of a "large white spot" and "grayish-white scabs" inside Irma's throat and mouth. In disbelief, Freud calls over a colleague, Dr. M., the leading mind of his medical circle, who also confirmed his discovery. Shortly thereafter, Freud's friends and colleagues, Otto and Leopold, join the examination. Of note is Freud's perception of both Otto and Leopold, as Freud considered Otto the more competent of the two physicians. As the group continued discussing Irma's condition, the final consensus indicated that Irma's condition was caused by an infection related to an injection she received with a dirty syringe that was administered by Otto.

The manifest content of the dream consisted of Freud diagnosing Irma's ailment (i.e., Freud discovered that Irma's illness was possibly related to an injection with a dirty syringe given to her by Otto, the colleague who informed him of her situation) and served the purpose of satisfying Freud's need of feeling competent. The latent content of the dream was related to Freud's sense of competency and the possible role he had played in her ailment. According to Freud's analysis of his dream,

> [t]he result of the dream is, that it is not I who am to blame for the pain which Irma is still suffering, but that Otto is to blame for it. Now Otto has annoyed me by his remarks about Irma's imperfect cure; the dream avenges me upon him, in that it turns the reproach upon himself. The dream acquitted me of responsibility for Irma's condition, as it refers this condition to other causes.
>
> (Freud, 1966, p. 205)

Based on Freud's analysis, his neurotic countertransference dream played two distinct roles: the re-establishment of Freud's competency, and wish-fulfillment based on the exculpating theme of his innocence as it relates to Irma's illness. According to Freud, "The dream represents a certain state of affairs, such as I might wish to exist; the content of the dream is thus the fulfillment of a wish; its motive is a wish" (p. 205). Although Freud's neurotic countertransference dream appeared to be a manifestation of his anxiety related to his competency and possible negative perception others may have of his ability, the distorted material within the dream (i.e., considering Leopold as more reliable than Otto, replacing Ana with her friend, and seeing Dr. M. as an "ignoramus") allowed him to become aware of and to externalize unwanted aspects of himself. In addition, the countertransference dream may have provided Freud with an opportunity to metabolize his repressed anger toward Irma. According to Myers (1987),

> [w]hile Freud does not discuss the dream from the point of view of countertransference, it seems clear from his tone of apology in writing of his anger towards Irma, that he had managed to effect some degree of resolution of his feelings towards his patient as the result of the analysis of this dream.
>
> (p. 37)

Winnicott (1994) and Searles (1958) also reported similar experiences related to a series of countertransference dreams that made them aware of their unconscious hate toward their patient. As a result of his dreams, Winnicott (1994) stated, "I have had a long series of these healing dreams which, although in many cases unpleasant, have each one of them marked my arrival at a new stage in emotional development" (p. 352). In other words, although neurotic countertransference dreams stem from analysts' neurosis and/or anxieties related to their patients, the analysis of such dreams provides analysts with information related to the therapeutic relationship in addition to fostering a reparative experience.

Projective Identification Countertransference Dreams

Projective identification countertransference dreams, as the category would suggest, are based on the Kleinian notion of projective identification. According to Klein (1946/1984), the concept of projective identification takes place when the patient splits a good or bad portion of the self and projects it onto an external object. As a result of the projection, the external object, the analysts in the case of treatment, experiences the feelings associated with the split as if it were their own. As the recipient of the patient's projection, the analyst gains an understanding of the patient's internal object relations. Projective identification countertransference dreams work in the same fashion, with the analyst's dream providing the analyst with an understanding of the patient's projected material. Although countertransference dreams commonly consist of neurotic distortions, Winnicott (1994) and Kron (1991) argue that certain aspects of the analyst's dream material consist of projected aspect of the patient's split or of their internal objects. Abramovitch and Lange (1994) stated,

> [t]he therapist's dreams may also reveal important aspects of the patient's unconscious and inner life, aspects of which the therapist is not sufficiently cognizant. Such dreams may, therefore, provide important and compensatory insight and therefore form a legitimate part of the therapeutic endeavor.
>
> (p. 106)

As a result of a countertransference dream, the analyst may become aware of certain aspects of the patient being projected onto them that requires metabolizing the patient's material. By doing so, the analyst will gain a greater understanding of the patient, and the patient will be able to tolerate the returned, and now conscious, metabolized material.

Another example of a projective identification countertransference dream is one shared in Waska's (2000) detailed recollection of an encounter with a former patient. Waska described his countertransference reaction toward his patient M. as "dislike and dread" in part due to her "irritating demeanor" (p. 35). Waska explained that his countertransference response was brought on by a sadomasochistic projective identification that involved a circular trading of "disdain and fear" between the two. In addition to their apparent dislike toward one another, Waska encountered frequent power struggles with the patient, and was commonly placed in the role of the rejected and abandoned while the client identified as the aggressor. The result was that Waska had feelings of fear and mistrust of the client as well as an "internally dead" feeling inside.

Throughout treatment, M. frequently mentioned her desire to terminate treatment and eventually terminated, an action Waska interpreted as an "interpersonal aspect of an intrapsychic repetition compulsion process in which she abandoned me much in the way, I believe, that she herself had felt chronically rejected" (Waska, 2000, p. 36). Shortly after being informed of her plan to terminate, Waska had a countertransference dream related to M. Within the dream, Waska attended a large rock concert and explored the surroundings of the venue. While walking through the crowd, Waska noticed an overweight female hippie he was able to convince to accompany him into a nearby cottage. A few points of interest related to the dream are that M. was a fan of rock music, and was best described as obese. While in the cottage, Waska murdered the woman by slashing her throat. He then disposed of her body. After blending into the crowd, Waska experienced a sense of fear over the possibility of being caught; however, he felt no remorse over what he had done.

According to Waska's analysis, M. projected onto (interpersonally) and into (intrapsychically) him her self-loathing and hatred toward her internal objects in addition to her fear of retaliation by those same objects, resulting in a circular interaction between Waska and M. that centered on fear and hostility. In the ideal situation, as it relates to projective identification, Ogden (1979) argues that

> [t]he projector fantasies ridding himself of an aspect of himself and putting that aspect into another person in a controlling way. Secondly, via the interpersonal interaction, the projector exerts pressure on the recipient of the projection to experience feelings that are congruent with the projection. Finally, the recipient psychologically processes the projection and makes a modified version available for re-internalization by the projector . . . one's projective fantasies impinge upon real external objects in a sequence of externalization and internalization.
>
> (p. 371)

Waska (2000) added,

> [t]he patient relates a specific unfinished psychic agenda. The psychotherapist must understand, modify, and interpret the patient's projections in a way that allows the patient to identify with them in a new light. The patient then identifies through both interpersonal and intrapsychic channels – the same channels through which the original projections emerged.
>
> (p. 37)

In other words, through projective identification, the patient is asking the analyst to accomplish what he or she was not able to achieve: the neutralizing of an overwhelming affect and in a way, to serve as an auxiliary ego function. Ideally, the analyst is able to understand, metabolize, and interpret the patient's unconscious material in order for the patient to internalize a detoxified object. However, due to Waska's difficulty in metabolizing M's projections, he became overwhelmed by the feelings associated with the projections and experienced a similar emotional response to that of M. Through his projective identification countertransference dream, Waska was able to metabolize the patient's "poisonous" projections "and partially master this malign force. In fact, I sought it out and actively did away with it, feeling the murder was a necessary evil" (p. 36). As a result of his dream, Waska was able to address his unconscious fantasies, which, in turn, allowed him to detoxify M's projections. Shortly thereafter, Waska became less standoffish and more accepting of M., leading to an interpersonal shift within the therapeutic relationship that eliminated, and, in a way, murdered the internal threat. This allowed M. to introject a modified and detoxified version of her projections without the fear of persecution.

Intersubjective Countertransference Dreams

Intersubjective countertransference dreams are viewed as an intricate part of treatment because of their ability to assist analysts in understanding the dynamics of the therapeutic relationship. Unlike neurotic and projective identification countertransference dreams that lean toward psychodynamic theory, writings focusing on intersubjective countertransference dreams implement a wide variety of theoretical approaches, including that of Jungian psychology (Kron, 1991). The conceptualization and analysis of such dream material focuses on the intersubjective process instead of the patient's history. In doing so, the dreams reveal important aspects of treatment the analyst was previously unaware of while also providing the analyst with an opportunity to resolve countertransference responses previously interfering with treatment (Kron, 1991; Abramovitch & Lange, 1994; Pollack-Gomolin, 2002).

According to Kron (1991), countertransference dreams, in particular intersubjective countertransference dreams, consist of more than simply the analyst's intrapsychic experience or the patient's projections onto the analyst. They primarily focus on the dynamics of the therapeutic relationship. Intersubjective countertransference dreams reflect the "meeting" between the patient and analyst and are associated with the dialogical dimension of the therapeutic relationship. The "meeting" takes place in what Kron called the "interhuman." Kron (1991) stated, "Emotions and fantasies have no interhuman meaning if they stay in the intrapsychic realm, but if they are brought out into the space 'between,' they can become meaningful" (p. 3). Although Kron uses the term *interhuman* to describe the interaction and space between the patient and analyst, she is actually referring to the transcendent function, the bridge that connects the conscious and unconscious processes of both the patient and the analyst, "signifying for the therapist the possibility of turning toward his patient and opening the way to dialogue between them" (Kron, 1991, p. 9). According to Jung (1958/1969), the trained analyst is able to "mediates the transcendent function for the patient, i.e., helps him to bring conscious and unconscious together and so arrive at a new attitude. In this function of the analyst lies one of the many important meanings of the transference" (p. 74). In other words, intersubjective countertransference dreams serve as a mechanism that allows the analyst to enter the transition space between the therapeutic dyad and communicate at an unconscious level within the transcendent function. Through this unconscious interaction, the analyst's dream highlights aspects of treatment and the therapeutic relationship of which the analyst was previously unaware. In addition, the unconscious interaction creates an arena to address and resolve their countertransference reactions.

In order to illustrate the workings of intersubjective countertransference dreams, Pollack-Gomolin's (2002) dream of Ms. H. and her interpretation of the dream will be examined in closer detail. Pollack-Gomolin described Ms. H. as a young woman who sought treatment as a result of her depressive symptoms. In addition, Ms. H reported being unhappy with her job, school, and romantic relationship, and attributed such difficulties and dissatisfaction to her painful upbringing, dysfunctional family, and previous abusive relationship. During the initial 7 months of treatment, Ms. H. focused mainly on her somatic symptoms during the first part of her sessions and concluded the beginning part of each session by stating that she had "now told me everything" (p. 59). Ms. H's expectation after each description of her "body talk" required Pollack-Gomolin to ask her diagnostic questions in the same fashion as the medical professionals she was consulting regarding her numerous physical ailments. Although Pollack-Gomolin found this request odd and confusing, she complied, and asked Ms. H. to be more descriptive of what she would like to be asked. As Pollack-Gomolin complied, Ms. H became more comfortable as sessions progressed and would commonly focus on her perceptions and dissatisfaction with others. Ms. H. described people as "intrusive, forever asking the wrong questions, angering her and invoking total indignation" (p. 59). As treatment progressed, Pollack-Gomolin began feeling similar to how Ms. H. described others – feeling incompetent and disconnected from Ms. H. In addition, Pollack-Gomolin began feeling a sense of hate toward Ms. H. as a result of her feeling "analytically impotent" (p. 59). Eight months into treatment, Pollack-Gomolin had a dream the night prior to their regularly scheduled session. During the dream, Pollack-Gomolin met Ms. H. in a "fancy" new office that also happened to be Pollack-Gomolin's personal apartment. The analytic couch was a sofa bed; however, only Pollack-Gomolin knew about that. Ms. H. was accompanied by a man and a young child. The identity of both was unknown to Pollack-Gomolin, but she wondered if the man was potentially Ms. H's boyfriend or ex-husband. Throughout the session, Pollack-Gomolin remained quiet and confused, and refrained from asking questions. Finally, she asked Ms. H. about the identity of the man whom she identified as her ex-husband. Pollack-Gomolin then inquired about the child's identity, a question Ms. H. answered by asking, "Didn't I tell you I had a child?" The following day during their scheduled session, Ms. H. began in her usual fashion by focusing on her physical ailments. As the session progressed, she began informing Pollack-Gomolin of her recent visit to her mother's house. While visiting her mother, she began looking through boxes of old pictures and mentioned seeing a picture of her ex-husband's child. As a result of her dream the previous night, Pollack-Gomolin was "completely dumbfounded." Similar to her dream, Pollack-Gomolin asked for clarification about Ms. H's ex-husband's child, to which she replied, "Didn't I tell you he had a child?"

By examining the manifest content of the dream in closer detail, the analytic setting being in the analyst's personal apartment symbolized the merger between the personal and analytic, or Ms. H's submersion into Pollack-Gomolin's unconscious space in what she described as "an evocative illustration of the narcissistic transference relationship and the therapeutic space where the unconscious conflicts of the analyst and patient resonate at latent levels of discovery and processing" (Pollack-Gomolin, 2002, p. 60). Through this unconscious interaction, Pollack-Gomolin became aware of the similarities between herself and Ms. H., both being private women who struggle connecting emotionally with others and who prefer to be alone, "arousing the analyst's like narcissistic tendency toward isolation and exclusion" (p. 60). In addition, Pollack-Gomolin mentioned sharing a similar sense of modesty, inhibitions, and fears as Ms. H., bringing to the forefront of treatment the transference/countertransference dynamic between the therapeutic dyad that focused on the potential consequence of not saying the right thing, being seen as inferior, and the fear of abandonment. In other words, Pollack-Gomolin was able to remove herself from what she called the mutuality of the dyad's dynamic tendencies, allowing her to view the collective "us" within the therapeutic relationship. In addition, Pollack-Gomolin interpreted the hideaway bed as a symbolic representation of their shared resistance to intimacy and touch, and the child as a representation of their inner child, with Ms. H. seeking Pollack-Gomolin's guidance to grow as an individual and move beyond the child within, and Pollack-Gomolin seeking to grow professionally. As a result of her dream, Pollack-Gomolin became aware of the dynamics of the therapeutic relationship as a whole, including the interfering nature of her resistance. In other words, Pollack-Gomolin's dream provided her with an entry into the transitional space or transcendent function, connecting the conscious and unconscious processes of the patent and analyst, leading to an understanding of the patient's transference in addition to the personal and professional growth of both members of the therapeutic dyad.

5 Countertransference From a Cognitive-Behavioral Approach

Historically, cognitive-behavioral approaches have focused very little on the phenomenon of countertransference. The lack of interest in countertransference within literature concerning cognitive-behavioral therapy may suggest that countertransference is not considered an important component of cognitive-behavioral treatment or that it simply does not occur when using such treatment modality (Gelso & Hayes, 2007). However, according to Gelso and Hayes (2007), this is simply untrue, as all therapists, "by virtue of their humanity, are prone to having their conflicts and vulnerabilities stimulated, by patients regardless of their theoretical orientation" (p. 52). Since cognitive-behavioral approaches tend to focus on technical factors as opposed to relational ones in order to promote change, countertransference is believed to play a smaller role in the therapeutic process and outcome of treatment in comparison to other treatment modalities (Gelso & Hayes, 2007). Nevertheless, this does not eliminate the role and effects countertransference can have on cognitive-behavioral-based treatment.

The basic premise behind countertransference is that it is predominantly a psychodynamic concept (Gelso & Hayes, 2007). Although deeply rooted in psychoanalytic theory, countertransference is a commonly occurring phenomenon within cognitive-behavioral treatment, leading to the expansion of cognitive-behavioral theories and concepts related to countertransference (Gelso & Hayes, 2007). As a way of separating countertransference from its psychodynamic origins, cognitive-behavioral theorists prefer to use language more appropriate to cognitive-behavioral theory (i.e., therapeutic belief system) when referring to countertransference (Rudd & Joiner, 1997; Gelso & Hayes, 2007). This is a necessary separation, as psychodynamic tenets are inconsistent with those of cognitive-behavioral therapy. Whereas psychodynamic approaches emphasize the importance of the alive and active unconscious inner world based on early relations and how past experiences influence future ones, cognitive-behavioral therapy stresses the importance of material close to the surface and relatively close to the present, focusing on the here and now as opposed to influences from the patient's past (Gelso & Hayes, 2007). Cognitive-behavioral techniques are also considered to be more standardized and formulaic as opposed to other approaches, making the role of therapist more of a "technician," with

DOI: 10.4324/9781003320180-6

the therapist's vulnerabilities and internal conflicts less relevant to treatment (Gelso & Hayes, 2007). Strupp (1958), however, emphasized the importance and role of the therapist, believing that therapeutic success was not based on technique alone, but on the method of delivery and factors associated with the therapist's personality as well. Strupp (1958) stated,

> In any case, it is clear that therapeutic techniques are not applied *in vacuo,* and that they are differentially affected by factors in the therapist's personality. His performance is determined – in part, at least – by the way in which he perceives the patient's behavior, interprets its meaning in the framework of his clinical experience *and* his own personality, and the way in which this meaning is reflected in his response. It is one of the peculiarities of the therapeutic situation that the therapist's interpersonal perceptions are immediately translated into action deliberately designed to effect a change in the patient's perceptions and behavior.
>
> (p. 35)

Goldfried and Davison (1994) added to the same idea by stating, "Any behavioral therapist who maintains that principles of learning and social influence are all one needs to know in order to bring about behavioral change is out of contact with clinical reality" (p. 55). Although cognitive-behavioral therapists view conditioning, reinforcement, and social influence as key components to patient problems, "the truly skillful behavioral therapist is one who can both conceptualize problems behaviorally and make the necessary translations so that he interacts in a warm and empathic manner with his client" (Goldfried & Davison, 1994, p. 56), meaning the effectiveness of treatment is enhanced by a positive relationship with the patient. In other words, cognitive-behavioral therapy consists of more than simply employing cognitive-behavioral techniques. It also includes therapists' methods of diagnosing, conceptualizing, and treating their patients. This for the most part is subjective and influenced by individual therapists' internal conflicts, again bringing us back to the inevitability of countertransference.

According to cognitive-behavioral theorists, countertransference is defined as "projections onto others of schemas derived from one's personal history" (Corsini, 2016, p. 1015). Ellis (2001) added by positing that countertransference originates from the therapist's irrational beliefs, automatic thoughts, scripts, and prototypes, making countertransference "the result of overgeneralized learning on behalf of the therapist" based on templates developed through the therapist's personal experiences (Gelso & Hayes, 2007, p. 56). Very similar to the way Freud (1912/1958) viewed transference as being caused by the development of "stereotype plates" based on personal experiences, cognitive behaviorists view countertransference as being caused by the same "stereotype plates," ultimately resulting in distorted views of the patient, and the therapist's inability to decipher between the patient and an individual from the past (Gelso & Hayes, 2007). Although countertransference can negatively impact cognitive-behavioral treatment as a result of the therapist's automatic thoughts, irrational beliefs, schemas, prototypes, and scripts, countertransference reactions may provide some insight into treatment. According to Gelso and Hayes (2007), countertransference reactions provide a possible reflection and behavioral sample of how the patient affects others, allowing the therapist to experience and observe their reaction to the patient's interpersonal dynamics. In other words, by examining and interpreting their emotional response to the patient, the therapist is able to understand the reaction of others interacting with the patient (Gelso & Hayes, 2007).

Most recently, the opinion of countertransference from a cognitive-behavioral perspective has expanded to consider the emotional response of the therapist as a fundamental component of treatment. Leahy (2001) stressed the importance of countertransference within cognitive-behavioral treatment, believing it was unavoidable regardless of how objective and technique driven the therapist may be. Given that countertransference is seen strictly as a psychodynamic tenet, Leahy (2001) focused on assimilating and implementing psychodynamic concepts within cognitive-behavioral approaches. According to Leahy (2001), "Psychodynamic concepts of transference, countertransference, and even ego defenses may be useful in helping us understand and change our patient's problems" (p. 5). By assimilating psychodynamic concepts into cognitive-behavioral approaches, in particular, the concept of countertransference, the therapist is able to gain a greater understanding of the patient's relationship with the therapist, and the therapist's response to the relationship. Through the exploration of countertransference, the therapist also becomes his or her own patient and gains insight into the patient's internal world by examining his or her own. Leahy (2001) stated,

> None of us is free from countertransference – nor should we be. To understand our own limitations, our own resistance to change, is to discover more about the patient and ourselves: as we learn about the how the patient's behavior affects our own countertransference, we are also learning about how the patient affects others.
>
> (p. 239)

In other words, therapists gain insight into patients' difficulties with abandoning old patterns and behaviors by exploring their personal struggles related to the same issue, as "both patient and therapist are patients" within the therapeutic relationship (Leahy, 2001, p. 5). In addition, the therapist is also able to experience how the patient affects others.

Prasko et al. (2010) shared similar views to Leahy (2001) and stressed the importance of countertransference, believing it occurred as the result of the therapist's response to the patient's transference. Although cognitive-behavioral treatment emphasizes technique and the use of psychopharmacology, the therapist's emotional response to the patient is unavoidable. As a result, Prasko et al. (2010) recommended the need for therapists to develop an understanding of their internal world and limitations. The expectation of cognitive-behavioral therapists is to have the ability to recognize, understand, and express their own emotions. By understanding their own limitations and resistances to change, therapists are able to gain insight not only about themselves but also about their patients, in particular, the therapist's response to the patient and how that is a possible reflection of how others experience the patient. Focusing strictly on the patient's behaviors allows therapists to avoid and compartmentalize their emotional response and personal problems, and in some cases displace their personal problems onto the patient. In other words, therapists become aware of their emotional responses as opposed to repressing them, while also reflecting on how such responses affect the therapeutic environment. This is a key aspect when examining countertransference from a cognitive-behavioral perspective, as the presence of countertransference suggests the presence of automatic thoughts on the part of the therapist (Prasko et al., 2010). However, focusing strictly on the patient's problems allows the therapist to neglect the presence of their countertransference while simultaneously projecting their personal problems and conflicts onto the patient (Prasko et al., 2010). In addition, the therapist's countertransference response may be a reflection of the treatment process for the patient. Through their ability to deal with and tolerate their countertransference responses, therapists are able to gain an understanding of their patients' experiences, leading to the progression of treatment.

Prasko et al. (2010) and Leahy (2001) identified a number of problems related to countertransference and how such problems can affect the progress of treatment. The identified issues are as follows:

- Ambivalence about using techniques because of fears of alienating the patient;
- Guilt or fear over the patient's anger;
- Feeling of inferiority when working with narcissistic patients;
- Discomfort if the patient is sexually attractive;
- Inability to set limits on sexually provocative or hostile patients;
- Overextending therapy sessions;
- Lack of assertion in collecting fees or enforcing policies;
- Inhibition in taking an adequate sexual history;
- Anger at patients who make phone calls between sessions;
- Catastrophizing the issue of hospitalizing a patient.

(Prasko et al., 2010, p. 194; Leahy, 2001, p. 241)

Such countertransference responses are commonly linked to the material presented by the patient in treatment; however, how does this relate to the therapist? Leahy (2001) reminds the therapist that as part of treatment, "you are not only applying techniques and conceptualizing problems, you are applying *yourself*" (p. 241). In other words, difficulties presented by the patient may activate vulnerabilities within the therapist related to the same difficulties.

According to Prasko et al. (2010) and Leahy (2001), automatic thought distortions play a key role in the development of countertransference. Commonly seen automatic thought distortions within psychotherapy include labeling, fortune telling, all-or-nothing thinking, personalizing, catastrophizing, shoulds, and over-generalizing (Prasko et al., 2010; Leahy, 2001). This occurs as a result of therapists applying themselves in addition to techniques and conceptualizing their patients' problems. Leahy (2001) stated,

> [w]hen patients present with issues such as abandonment, dependency, devaluation, demandingness, sexual preoccupation, abuse, betrayal, or exploitation of others, they may arouse your own feelings and vulnerabilities about these issues. Hiding behind the techniques of cognitive therapy or dismissing the patient with a label ("She's a borderline") will inadvertently sabotage therapy. Perhaps some patients are exquisitely tuned to the countertransference in the therapist – perhaps they can "read" the therapist's vulnerabilities. But we cannot make the countertransference go away simply because we might wish it did not affect the treatment.
>
> (p. 241)

This, however, allows for the use of countertransference as a tool to assist patients with their difficulties, as it provides the therapist with a glimpse and experience of the "real world effects" patients have outside of the therapeutic relationship (Leahy, 2001, p. 241). For instance, if patients devalue therapists, they may also devalue others. This can be useful not only in diagnosing the patients but also in helping them understand how their behaviors affect others, and how such modes of interaction were developed, with the ultimate goal being assisting the patient in developing a more effective method of interacting and relating to others in therapy.

In addition to the therapist's automatic thoughts and distortions, schemas also play a significant role in countertransference reactions (Prasko et al., 2010; Leahy, 2001). In the same fashion as schemas lead to resistance for the patient within treatment, the same can occur for the therapist in the form of countertransference. Although there are a number of different schemas that could activate the therapist as a result of the patient, Prasko et al. (2010) and Leahy (2001) warn against four of the most common maladaptive schemas and how they can influence the course of treatment.

Demanding Standards Schema

The demanding standards schema is commonly seen with perfectionistic and obsessive-compulsive therapists. In such scenarios, the perfectionistic and obsessive-compulsive therapist views the patient as lazy and irresponsible, and considers the expression of emotions as fruitless, unnecessary, and devastating to treatment (Prasko et al., 2010). As a result, such therapists encounter difficulties in empathizing and expressing warmth toward their patients. The emphasis of treatment becomes efficiency, logic, and rationality as opposed to the expression of the patient's emotional needs, leading to the patient's emotional turmoil being overlooked. In other words, the perfectionistic and obsessive-compulsive therapist creates unrealistic expectations not only for the patient but for themselves as well (Leahy, 2001). Therapists encountered with such issues may attempt to overcompensate for their feelings of inadequacy by demanding and expecting perfection from themselves and their patients. Because the patient may not be able to keep up with the demanding therapist's expectations, the patient may interpret this as a failure. The patient is attempting to move at the therapist's pace instead of moving forward at his or her own pace (Leahy, 2001). In addition, a perfectionistic and obsessive-compulsive therapist may attempt to deal with their feelings of incompetence by avoiding working with difficult patients or by raising the expectation set for the patient (Prasko et al., 2010).

Abandonment Schema

According to Leahy (2001), abandonment is another common schema that plays a role in countertransference. Under such circumstances, the therapist will experience feelings of concern over the possibility of the patient prematurely leaving treatment, leading to lack of confrontation by the therapist, even when appropriate. The therapist will perceive the termination of treatment as a personal rejection (Leahy, 2001). The fear of abandonment may be a reflection of attachment issues on the part of the therapist, as the therapist may present as clingy by being overly protective of the patient through excessive caretaking, or prevent and avoid the possibility of entering a meaningful therapeutic relationship with the patient as a way of preventing the anticipated and inevitable abandonment by the patient. The excessive caretaking therapist will shield and protect the patient from experiencing difficult situations and will take the patient's problems as his or her own (Leahy, 2001). In contrast, the attachment avoidant therapist uses such strategy to avoid the possibility and threat of abandonment. The attachment avoidant therapist will see the patient simply as a collection of symptoms and will avoid the patient's more meaningful personal issues by focusing on superficial techniques, reducing the likelihood of an attachment and abandonment. In such circumstances, the therapist will avoid difficult topics or using anxiety-provoking interventions. In addition, the avoidant therapist will interpret the patient's resistance as a personal rejection and potential abandonment by the patient (Prasko et al., 2010). To avoid the rejection and potential abandonment, the therapist will avoid any form of confrontation with the patient. This avoidance includes the choice of not confronting the patient's irrational beliefs or self-destructive behaviors, compromising the therapist's professionalism as a way of keeping the patient interested and involved in treatment while simultaneously preventing the abandonment that is feared (Prasko et al., 2010).

Special, Superior Person Schema

According to Prasko et al. (2010) and Leahy (2001), this specific schema refers to the narcissistic therapist, as such a therapist views therapy as an opportunity to shine and show off his or her abilities as a superior therapist. The narcissistic therapist feels an entitlement toward the patient and expects the patient's cooperation within treatment. Because the narcissistic therapist views himself or herself as superior to others, he or she tends to have boundary issues, as boundaries, like any other rules, do not apply to the narcissist (Leahy, 2001). In addition, the narcissistic therapist may attempt to validate his or her image by vilifying previously failed therapeutic relationships and pinpointing how other therapists have failed the patient.

The narcissistic therapist's interest in the patient is conditional and is dependent on the patient's improvement. The narcissistic therapist tends to use the patient as a way of legitimatizing the therapist's own greatness (Prasko et al., 2010). The lack of improvement in a patient raises doubt within the therapist, as the lack of improvement raises doubt about the therapist's ability and greatness. Instead of empathizing with the patient for the lack of improvement, the therapist will lose interest in the patient and express anger toward him or her (Leahy, 2001). The therapist will attack the patient by questioning his or her desire to improve while also taking the lack of improvement as a personal attack, one that questions the therapist's superiority and makes him or her no different than the therapists he or she previously vilified.

Narcissistic therapists tend to use the three defenses commonly seen within narcissists: idealization, devaluation, and distancing. Narcissistic therapists may idealize a patient, in particular, those they deem attractive and successful, as a way of validating their perception and self-worth, reveling in their patient's success. However, the act of idealizing serves as a compensatory feeling from the true feeling of envy the therapist may be experiencing as a result of the patient's perceived success (Leahy, 2001). If the patient does not live up to the therapist's idealization and expectations as treatment progresses, the narcissistic therapist may turn on the patient by devaluing them in addition to ridiculing their situation and way of thinking. The patient's resistance is seen as a failure on behalf of the patient as opposed to an opportunity of working with the patient's vulnerabilities. The narcissistic therapist will see this as proof of the patient's inability to be helped instead of an indication of the therapist's own shortcomings resulting from his or her own countertransference. As a result of the perceived shortcomings on behalf of the patient, the narcissistic therapist will begin to distance himself or herself from the patient. The therapist sees the patient as someone who failed him or her and loses interest while simultaneously showing little empathy or authentic validation toward the patient (Prasko et al., 2010). Such actions by the narcissistic therapist lead to a profound negative effect on the patient, as the patient will consider the failed therapeutic relationship as an affirmation that others cannot be trusted or that they cannot be understood.

Need for Approval Schema

The need for approval is characteristic of the people-pleasing therapist. Such therapists aim at making patients feel good regardless of their situation and have difficulties with patients expressing any form of anger or disappointment (Leahy, 2001). The pleasing therapist may be skillful at showing empathy, resulting in the patient feeling valued and understood; however, this may prevent the therapist from seeing or acknowledging the patient's anger and frustration, as the pleasing therapist perceives the patient's anger as a reflection of the therapist's own failure and will purposefully avoid conflict (Prasko et al., 2010). The pleasing therapist will also avoid topics considered too difficult for the patient as a way of avoiding conflict with the patient. By doing so, the therapist is communicating with the patient that he or she either approves of the patient's maladaptive behaviors or simply does not care about them.

In addition to the four identified schemas, Leahy (2001) also identifies two additional schemas: the excessive self-sacrifice schema and the autonomy schema. According to Leahy (2001), the self-sacrificing therapist tends to prioritize the needs of the patient at the expense of the therapist's own; however, the gratification for the therapist lies in the therapist feeling needed by the patient. Under such circumstances, the therapist hinders the therapeutic relationship by serving as a poor role model to the patient and blurring professional boundaries. In addition, the self-sacrificing therapist may be reluctant to challenge the patient out of fear of how the patient will respond. Therapists with a strong sense of autonomy tend to experience difficulties as well, in particular, with the patient's emotional expressions, demands for extra attention, and refusal to comply with assigned tasks (Leahy, 2001). Therapists experiencing this form of countertransference develop an expectation of the patient and their ability to handle situations independently.

Due to the potential affect of countertransference on the therapeutic relationship, Prasko et al. (2010) encourage therapists to be aware of their response to the patient as a way of reducing the possibility of the therapist acting out and retaliating against the patient. Similar to the way the therapist is expected to tend to the patient's emotional responses, therapists are also expected to do the same as it relates to emotional response to the content within sessions. By doing so, the therapist is able to reflect on both positive and negative reactions, and determine how much of their response is related to their own personal experiences or to their existing opinions of the content being covered in treatment.

Although countertransference from a cognitive-behavioral perspective is occasionally seen as a possible aid to treatment, as it has the potential of providing the therapist with a view of how their behavior affects others, its role continues to be ambiguous. Literature continues to minimize the significance of the therapist's internal experience, making his or her thoughts, feelings, and perceptions of the patient irrelevant (Gelso & Hayes, 2007). Nevertheless, countertransference is brought on by these internal experiences, leading to a distorted view of the patient, and selective attention to patient material depending on how it related to the therapist (McClure & Hodge, 1987). Gelso and Hayes (2007) argue that by minimizing the internal experience of the therapist, cognitive-behavioral approaches inadvertently promote countertransference responses and behaviors.

Clinical Case Example – Perfectly Imperfect

Christian reached out to ML for therapy after the unexpected passing of his wife. Christian described their relationship as loving and focused on the feelings of loss early in treatment. Although Christian denied having any anger or negative emotions toward his wife, he acknowledged struggling with having to independently take care of their 3-year-old son and the family's debt.

As treatment progressed, ML noticed that he developed a "special liking" toward Christian and began looking forward to their sessions. He also noticed that his treatment approach was out of character, focusing on the process of grief and loss while also allowing Christian to talk about "my wonderful wife." Although ML believed it was important for Christian to process and grieve the loss of his wife, he found himself being passive instead of challenging Christian's false beliefs and irrational thoughts. Their interactions were more conversational and similar to a conversation between friends instead of an exchange between therapist and client.

After reflecting on his approach, ML encouraged the discussion of more difficult topics. Christian described his upbringing as "wonderful" and his parents as "loving and supportive." Christian met his wife in college and described her as "flawless" as he found her extremely attractive. He also appreciated her confidence and career aspirations. Christian described his son as "a joy" but acknowledged feelings of sadness related to his son having to grow up without his mother. Although Christian characterized his relationship with his wife as ideal, he admits that she was experiencing some depression prior to her passing after the tragic death of her mother.

Over time, ML recognized the grief and loss experienced by Christian. However, he also recognized the idealization of his family and the core belief that everything needed to be perfect, including himself. As a result, Christian felt that he was only lovable when he and his situation were perfect. This also became noticeable in treatment as Christian would frequently praise ML and expressed how grateful he was to be working with him. While ML explored his countertransference response toward Christian, ML became aware that he was conspiring with him and his expectations of perfection as it related to relationships. ML wanted to be the perfect therapist and the one to care for and rescue Christian. After further self-exploration, ML realized that his countertransference response was brought on by his ongoing need for approval and the idealization and unexpected loss of his own mother. ML acknowledged difficulties addressing loss, making it challenging to address painful and uncomfortable experiences with Christian. ML had not only identified with Christian's loss but he was also seeking Christian's approval and acting out his personal need to please others. In more specific terms, ML's countertransference response was caused by the activation of his need for approval schema. As a result, ML was fearful of being abandoned and instead focused on pleasing, caring for, and rescuing Christian. ML's attempt to care for and rescue Christian was, in fact, an attempt to rescue himself and fulfill his need for approval.

After becoming aware of the meaning of his countertransference response toward Christian, ML was able to re-establish his role as therapist. From that point forward, ML and Christian addressed difficult issues such as his core belief of being unlovable and the assumption of needing to be perfect to be worthy of love. In addition, ML and Christian explored Christian's need to avoid difficult interactions with others. Over the remaining course of treatment, Christian discussed his feelings toward his wife, including her perceived selfishness and situations where she disappointed him. He also expressed his anger toward her for being under the influence of alcohol during the car accident that resulted in her death. Although Christian acknowledged difficulties in being vulnerable and discussing his emotions, he was able to gain a deeper understanding of his core beliefs and was able to integrate a greater sense of balance into his life.

6 Humanistic Psychology and Countertransference

Similar to cognitive-behavioral literature, humanistic psychology seldom mentions the phenomenon of countertransference. The infrequent focus on countertransference, however, is not to say that the therapist's internal conflicts and vulnerabilities are irrelevant and instead are a result of semantics (Gelso & Hayes, 2007). Bugental (1978), for example, provides a description of what appears to be countertransference; however, he refrains from terming the phenomenon being described. According to Bugental (1978), "Each therapist has a unique pattern of open receptivity, areas of partial interference in which it is harder for the client's experiences to get through, and areas of relevant or absolute blindness" (p. 42). In addition, Bugental stated:

> The ideal psychotherapist is one who seeks to get and keep his or her act together. The ideal therapist recognizes that the emotions, conflicts, biases, and anxieties of the therapist's own life inevitably have their effects on the client's life, and this is not an idle recognition. Thus the ideal therapist accepts the responsibility for continuing self-monitoring to reduce the untoward impact of the therapist's distresses on the client.
>
> (p. 34)

Again, Bugental does not specifically mention countertransference by name; however, the specifics described are in fact countertransference. In addition, Bugental warns against the possible influence the therapist's emotional response can have on the therapeutic relationship, another factor associated with countertransference.

Meador and Rogers (1984) also discuss what appears to be countertransference; however, they do so using terminology associated with humanistic psychology. Meador and Rogers (1984) describe it in the following manner:

> Genuineness and congruence is the basic ability of the therapist to read his own inner experiencing and to allow the quality of his inner experiencing to be apparent in the therapeutic relationship. That precludes his playing a role or presenting a facade. His words are consonant with his experiencing. He follows himself transparently. He follows the changing flow of his own

DOI: 10.4324/9781003320180-7

feelings and presents himself transparently. He attempts to be fully present to this client; he is himself. . . . The therapist, in the fullness of his own person, tries to immerse himself in the feeling world of his client to experience that world within himself. His understanding comes out of his own inner experiencing of his client's feelings, using his own inner processes of awareness for a referent. He actively experiences not only the client's feelings, but also his own inner response to this feeling.

(p. 143)

In other words, Meador and Rogers (1984) felt the need for the therapists to submerge themselves in patients' experience, to become one with them, or as Yalom called it, to become "fellow travelers" with patients, and having a shared experience with them (Yalom, 2002). Bugental (1987) added:

Even more dismaying is the frequent lack of attention to therapist presence and the encouragement of "objectivity" and "therapeutic detachment." Indeed, there are those who take the attitude that the full presence of the therapist is a form of countertransference! "Therapeutic detachment," standing at an aseptic distance from the client has been – and for some still is – an ideal, counter therapeutic as it is. . . . I believe that the new paradigm – for psychotherapy, for psychology, for science, for society, for our times – is (and must be) recognizing the centrality of subjectivity.

(p. 47)

Unlike his previous writings, Bugental mentions countertransference by name and stresses the important role it plays within treatment. In addition, although Bugental encourages the need for a paradigm shift focusing on the subjective experience of the therapist versus the need for objectivity, the humanistic view on countertransference remained the same and semantics continued to be an issue.

In addition to semantics playing a role in the lack of countertransference discussions within humanistic psychology, countertransference is counterintuitive to the basic tenets of humanistic psychology. According to Gelso and Hayes (2007), "one of the fundamental humanistic tenets is the belief in the inherent goodness of human beings. The natural human tendency is considered to be toward health and development. By extension, one's inner experience largely is to be trusted" (pp. 64–65). This stance negates the negative qualities of the therapist, minimizing unresolved conflicts of the therapist commonly associated with countertransference. In addition, humanistic psychology does not see the therapist's thoughts and feelings as countertransference distortions, but instead as reality-based views of the patient. In other words, countertransference becomes nonexistent, fades into the background, and is superseded by the therapist's respect and connection with the patient (Gelso & Hayes, 2007; Meador & Rogers, 1982).

Although countertransference does not play a prominent role in humanistic psychology, the phenomenon is still inevitable and may hinder the prospering of psychotherapeutic progress and relationships. As mentioned by Rogers (2007), six necessary conditions must exist within a therapeutic relationship in order to promote change. They are as follows:

1. Two persons are in psychological contact.
2. The first, whom we shall term the client, is in a state of incongruence, being vulnerable or anxious.
3. The second person, whom we shall term the therapist, is congruent or integrated into the relationship.
4. The therapist experiences unconditional positive regard for the client.
5. The therapist experiences an empathic understanding of the client's internal frame of reference and endeavors to communicate this experience to the client.
6. The communication to the client of the therapist's empathic understanding and unconditional positive regard is to a minimal degree achieved. (Rogers, p. 241)

Since a humanistic approach focuses on the therapist trusting his or her own inner experience and bringing personal experience into treatment, it is impossible for the therapist to negate and ignore their unresolved issues and internal conflicts. Countertransference may inhibit the therapist's ability to remain authentic and congruent, leading to undesirable emotional responses such as anger and despair. According to Rogers (2007), a therapist is expected to be "a congruent, genuine, integrated person. It means that within the relationship he is freely and deeply himself, with his actual experience accurately represented by his awareness of himself" (p. 242). As a result, therapists are expected to behave in a manner that reflects or is congruent with their feelings, something Rogers encouraged. Rogers (1961) stated:

> It has made it seem to me that the most basic learning for anyone who hopes to establish any kind of helping relationship is that it is safe to be transparently real. If in a given relationship I am reasonably congruent, if no feelings relevant to the relationship are hidden either to me or the other person, then I can be almost sure that the relationship will be a helpful one.
> (p. 51)

However, this can become a complex ordeal, in particular, if the emotions experienced by the therapist are negative in nature. Although a humanistic approach requires congruency on behalf of the therapist, self-disclosure should not be taken lightly, as it can damage the therapeutic relation and have a hurtful impact on the patient. According to Curtis (1981), if a therapist uses self-disclosure

> As part of a spontaneous reaction to the patient, it may be viewed as an unidentified form of countertransference; this is observed when the

therapist's self-disclosing remarks serve to mitigate anxiety or some other affective state (e.g., hostility or guilt) which maintains a repression in response to unconscious material re-stimulated by the patient.

(p. 500)

The therapist cannot simply self-disclose without calculating the associated risk and possibility of hurting or harming the patient. When necessary, it is important for the therapist to sacrifice openness if it is in the best interest of the patient.

In addition to affecting the therapist's ability to remain congruent, countertransference can also be an impediment to the therapist's ability to provide unconditional positive regard to the patient. According to Gelso and Hayes (2007), countertransference reactions are perceived as threats, making it difficult to have unconditional positive regard for an individual who is seen as a danger. Additionally, by provoking the activation of unresolved conflicts, the therapist may develop a sense of resentment, resulting in the therapist acting in a defensive and judgmental manner. With countertransference being seen as a potential threat, the therapist goes into self-preservation mode. However, this also affects the therapist's ability to empathize with the patient, with the therapist beginning to focus on themselves as a way of self-preservation instead of the patient (Gelso & Hayes, 2007). Whether the therapist is over- or under-identifying with the patient, the countertransference experience activated his or her unresolved conflicts.

Clinical Case Example – The Fearful Bully

Jessica reached out to CJ at the suggestion of a close friend to address ongoing interpersonal conflict with loved ones and friends. Jessica was a married woman in her late thirties and a mother of two children, with her oldest being from a previous relationship. CJ described Jessica as aggressive and someone who lacked insight into her impact on others. Although Jessica participated in sessions, CJ acknowledged difficulties working with Jessica due to the "constant digs" she made toward her. As a result, CJ frequently found herself angry and frustrated with Jessica. In addition, CJ acknowledged feeling conflicted as a therapist practicing from a humanistic approach. CJ believed she might be experiencing a countertransference reaction to Jessica; however, according to theory, countertransference was counterintuitive to the basic tenets of humanistic psychology. In theory, CJ was expected to trust her inner experience as it reflected a reality-based view of the client. However, this experience was different due to the emotional charge she experienced in sessions. As a result, CJ questioned her authenticity, genuineness, and congruency early in treatment. Three months into treatment, CJ felt attacked by Jessica after an intense emotional session. CJ described Jessica's behavior as "mean, belittling, and aggressive." Before the end of session, Jessica smiled at CJ and asked if she was mad at her, appearing proud of the anger she may have provoked in CJ.

Although CJ was feeling intense anger toward Jessica, she instead focused on the fear brought on by Jessica and the sensation of feeling bullied. Jessica was astonished by CJ's disclosure as she was accustomed to causing anger in others. Jessica sat quietly on the couch and began crying. The fear experienced by CJ and Jessica's need to bully others symbolized Jessica's repressed fear and anxiety related to feeling inferior after her husband's infidelities. Jessica felt a sense of control that ensured her self-preservation by bullying others. In addition, CJ's disclosure provided Jessica with insight into how she impacts and affects others while also gaining insight into understanding her relationship and response to fear. Although CJ went against the basic premise of humanistic psychology, her countertransference reaction and disclosure allowed Jessica to gain a deeper understanding of her behavior while also connecting with the emotional anguish of her husband's infidelities.

7 Transtheoretical Definition of Countertransference

Countertransference has been a controversial concept since its inception and introduction by Freud in the early 1900s. Its definition has evolved and continues to do so over time, commonly being depicted as a potential positive or negative within a therapeutic encounter, or by looking at its potential effect toward the therapeutic relationship. There appears to be no single, clear-cut, transtheoretical definition. For the purpose of this book, an interpretive inquiry was conducted as a way of gaining a deeper and more comprehensive understanding of the psychological meanings and descriptions of countertransference. Through the use of hermeneutics, a series of selected writings/texts related to countertransference was interpreted as a way of allowing the researcher/interpreter to become "part of this circle moving repeatedly between interpretations of parts of the text and interpretations of the whole text, representing an emerging understanding of the phenomenon" (Paterson & Higgs, 2005, p. 343). Like the messenger-god Hermes, the interpreter serves as a bridge between the language of two worlds and brings "what is foreign, strange, or unintelligible into the medium of one's own language" (Palmer, 1969, p. 27). Palmer (1969) added:

> Like the god Hermes, the translator mediates between one world and another. The act of translation is not a simple mechanical matter of synonym-finding, as the ludicrous products of translation machines make only too clear, for the translator is mediating between two different worlds.
>
> (p. 27)

Unlike other qualitative research methods, hermeneutics, in particular, philosophical hermeneutics, looks at the lived experience of the interpreter "as they attune themselves towards the ontological nature of phenomenon while learning to 'see' pre-reflective, taken-for-granted, and essential understandings through the lens of their always already pre-understandings and prejudices" (Kafle, 2011, p. 188). Hermeneutic interpretation then becomes possible as a result of the relationship between the interpreter and the text, and their immersion into the work.

According to Packer and Addison (1989), "When we try to study some new thing we are always thrown into it" (p. 33). In other words, we must have a

DOI: 10.4324/9781003320180-8

point of entry to enter the hermeneutic circle of interpretation. My point of entry developed as a result of my personal experience related to countertransference, which set the foundation for understanding through my preexisting fore-structures, preconceptions, and experiences related to the phenomenon. Or, as Romanyshyn (2007) would argue, my entry into the hermeneutic circle resulted from my book topic choosing me as opposed to me choosing my topic through my unconscious complexes and personal struggles with countertransference. This exchange required me to relinquish my claim to the work, in addition to becoming a conduit of sorts by providing the research with a voice not only to be heard but also for it to develop a life of its own by using the past as a way of understanding the future. For the purpose of this book, the initial inquiry, or the launching into the forward arc of the hermeneutic circle, began with the question "What is countertransference?" in an attempt to discover a transtheoretical definition of countertransference, a concept that continues to elude the field of psychology as a result of definitions varying largely based on theoretical orientations. While attempting to define the concept of countertransference, additional points of inquiry emerged: What is pathological countertransference? How does pathological countertransference develop? How do analysts separate themselves from the patient's experience? What should analysts do to prevent their countertransference response from interfering with treatment? Although this chapter will focus on answering these questions using a neutral approach from a theoretical standpoint, countertransference is a concept based on psychodynamic theory, making it nearly impossible to eliminate psychodynamic tenets. As a result, psychodynamic terminology, in particular, that of object relations, will be observed throughout this chapter.

Although a philosophical hermeneutic approach was used for the basis of this book, the interpretation process implemented a phenomenological frame of mind to interpret the material. My experience through the hermeneutic circle did not introduce me to a number of different texts to examine and reinterpret, but instead it brought back to life some of the most influential minds of psychology. As a result of such an approach, I had the pleasure of "interviewing" the likes of Sigmund Freud, Carl Jung, Heinrich Racker, and Melanie Klein, to name a few. Through the "interview" process, each "interview" was examined as its own part and then united with the other "interviews" in order to understand the phenomenon of countertransference as a whole. Through the reciprocal interaction between "interviews" and the concept of countertransference as a whole, meaning-making and understanding became possible, ultimately leading to a clearer and universal understanding of countertransference.

What Is Countertransference?

The definition of countertransference varies across theoretical approaches to treatment; however, for the purpose of this book, countertransference will be defined as a spectrum of possible emotional responses on the part of the analyst, resulting from the psychic interaction between the conscious and unconscious processes of the patient and analyst. In addition, the analyst's emotional response is a direct correlation to the patient's transference. Given that countertransference manifestations will be examined within a spectrum of possibilities, emotional responses will consist of both positive and negative responses, including neurotic responses on the part of the analyst, and all possibilities in between.

Countertransference is a co-constructed, two-person phenomenon that occurs between the patient and analyst (Jung, 1935/1970; Heimann, 1950; Little, 1981; Racker, 1988; Aron, 1993; Leahy, 2001; Gelso & Hayes, 2007). Countertransference represents the "psychological symbiosis" between two personalities, or in other words, the interaction between the conscious and unconscious processes of the patient and analyst (Racker, 1988, p. 172). As Jung (1935/1970) argued, every individual represents a psychic system capable of affecting and interacting with other psychic systems. When such interactions occur, the prime result is a back-and-forth interaction resulting in the mutual influencing of the psychic systems involved. Through the exchange, the patient and the analyst experience a psychological connectedness resulting in a shared space that allows for the patient and the analyst to identify with each other through a shared experience (Jung, 1971; Leahy, 2001). The shared experience allows analysts to immerse themselves within the patient's emotional experience, becoming "fellow travelers" with their patients while simultaneously experiencing the world of their patients (Yalom, 2002). Aron (1998) writes,

> [i]n the course of a psychoanalytic journey, patient and analyst (while generally not literally touching each other's bodies) come to share a psychoanalytic skin-ego or psychoanalytic breathing ego. Within the fluid exchange of interpretive squiggles and mutual associations between patient and analyst, the question of whose idea that was, patient's or analyst's, who thought of this or that, is often not answerable. Gradually, patient and analyst mutually regulate each other's behaviors, enactments, and states of consciousness such that each gets under the other's skin, each reaches into the other's guts, each is breathed in and absorbed by the other. For a while, patient and analyst share a jointly created skin-ego/breathing self.
> (pp. 25–26)

In other words, as a result of the shared experience, an opportunity for healing and growth presents itself through the psychic interaction for those systems involved, leading to a greater understanding of the patient (Machtiger, 1982).

When examining the co-construction of countertransference, the phenomenon can be described by using alchemy as a metaphorical explanation to illustrate the interaction between the patient and analyst. For example, if we look at the basic premise of alchemy, the main goal of the alchemist was to combine chemical substances in hopes of activating a transformation within the substances leading to the discovery of a new chemical compound, in particular, the ability to transform metals into gold (Jung, 1946/1970; Redgrove, 1997;

Martin, 2001). The unconscious interaction within psychotherapy works in a similar fashion, with the analyst serving the function of the alchemist and the personalities of the therapeutic dyad representing the combination of chemical substances. The unconscious interactions between personalities also represent the transference/countertransference dynamic within treatment. Similar to the chemical interaction between substances, if an interaction occurs between personalities, a unification between personalities will take place, resulting in the transformation of both personalities involved (Jung, 1931/1970). For instance, if we look at Figure 7.1, we can see the conscious and unconscious interaction between the patient and analyst, and how the exchange takes place within the therapeutic setting. The image is a representation of the clinical setting or alchemical vessel where the mutual influencing takes place. The male and

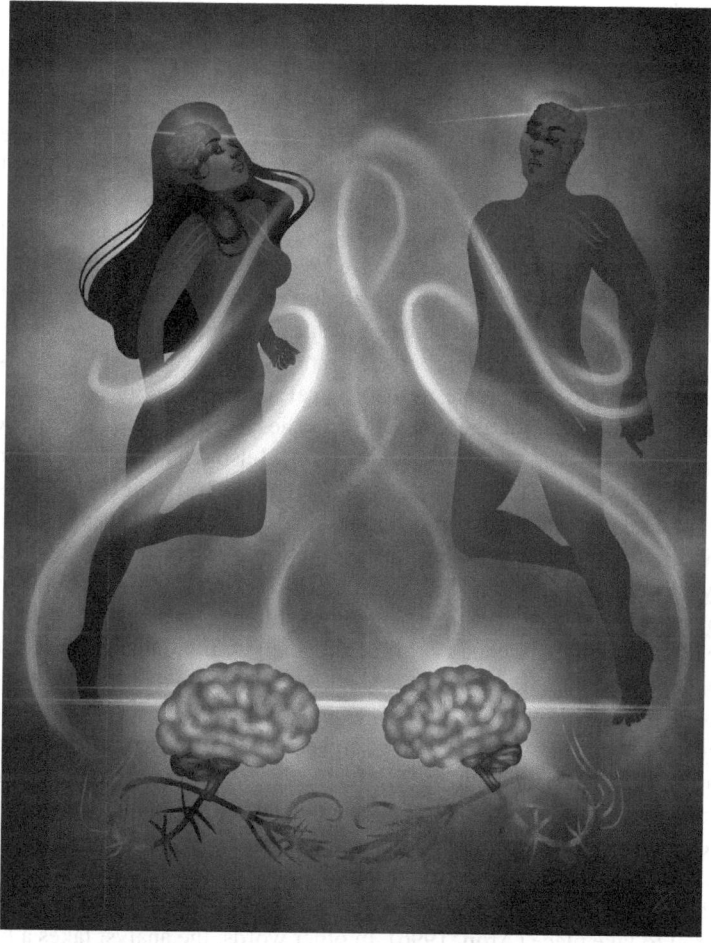

Figure 7.1 The psychic exchange, by A. Diffin, 2019

female images represent the analyst and patient as individuals. While on their own, the patient and analyst symbolize an individual psychic system, a separate and independent system of its own. The energy/light exiting each individual is a representation of the conscious and unconscious material of each independent psychic system. Throughout treatment, the material of each individual psychic system begins mixing within the alchemical vessel, leading to the psychic interaction, or mutual influencing between the psychic systems as shown in the image. As the psychic interaction continues, the newly discovered "element" emerges and circulates itself into each individual system, influencing and changing the individual psychic system as a whole. This is an ongoing process throughout treatment reminiscent of the hermeneutic circle, an ongoing mutual influencing resulting in a changed psychic system mirroring the discovery of new meaning through the reinterpretation of text. Countertransference is therefore a shared and lived experience between the patient and analyst.

The phenomenon of countertransference consists of the analyst's conscious and unconscious response to the patient's transference (Jung, 1931/1970; Little, 1981). Since transference is based on projections of the patient's past, or internal representations of the patient's past, the analyst's unconscious is activated by the patient's projections of such experiences, resulting in a counterprojection on the part of the analyst (Jung, 1931/1970; Racker, 1988). As Meier (1959) stated, "It may be assumed that the 'catching' of projections by a 'hook' cannot be without effects on the carrier, and that a counter-effect will not be lacking" (p. 23). Given that projections are based on the previous experiences of the patient and countertransference being analogous to transference, countertransference is therefore the fusion between the past and present, the conscious with the unconscious, a connection between fantasy and reality, and a representation of the analyst's complete psychological response and/or attitude toward the patient influenced by the analyst's fantasies, reality, and past experiences (Langs, 1976; Racker, 1988; Winnicott, 1994; Gelso & Hayes, 2007). Through psychotherapy, the transference/countertransference dynamic develops as a result of a relationship between two individuals, with the nurturing and growth within the relationship allowing for an emotional response on the part of the analyst to occur (Heimann, 1950; Little, 1981; Aron, 1996). In other words, countertransference is more than simply transference on the part of the analyst. Instead, countertransference is part of the analytic relationship co-created by the patient in conjunction with the analyst, a process initiated within the patient, although expanded by and within the analyst's unconscious. As a result, countertransference consists of all feelings and emotions experienced by the analyst toward the patient (Heimann, 1950, Machtiger, 1982). In addition, the circular interaction resulting from the transference/countertransference dynamic leads to the regulation of each individual's state of consciousness, moving regression from the individual's state of mind into the psychic space between the patient and analyst, allowing for the interpretation and analysis of the unconscious material to take place (Aron, 1996). In other words, the analyst takes a liminal position between consciousness and the unconscious in what Jung called the transcendent function, or the analytic third, as Ogden termed it (Miller, 2004). Returning to the alchemy or psychic exchange image, this liminal space serves as a container of sorts within the alchemical vessel that exists within the therapeutic setting.

According to Agnel (1992), the transcendent function, or the analytic third, serves as a "bridge between two worlds" (p. 105). Similar to the role of the messenger-god Hermes, who served as a bridge between the world of mortal man and the Gods, the analyst serves as a bridge connecting the unconscious realm with the conscious one, making what was once beyond human comprehension into something human intelligence could grasp and understand. Like Hermes, who had the ability to access multiple meanings or cross multiple boundaries, the analyst is able to access multiple levels of consciousness simultaneously, an in-betweenness that allows for the conscious and unconscious processes of the patient and analyst to interact in an alchemical-type fashion. For Jung, the psychic interaction was a mutual transaction between the analyst and patient, and is a prime example of the transference/countertransference dynamic within treatment (Carter, 2010). Comparable to the anticipated galactic collision between the Milky Way and Andromeda (Cox & Loeb, 2008; Park, 2018), the personalities of the patient and analyst collide within the transcendent function, leading to an interaction and a unification of sorts, that provides the analyst with an understanding of the patient's unconscious material. As a result of the co-constructed phenomenon, the analyst's conscious and unconscious responses to the real or imagined perception of the patient are used as a way of gaining an understanding of the interpersonal relationship between the patient and the analyst. The sum of these parts depicts the psychic reality of the analyst, a reality created through a dialectic process between two individuals, resulting in reciprocal or mutual influencing between the individuals involved (Jung, 1968a). As a result of this relationship, the emergence of the transcendent function takes place, providing the patient and analyst with the ability to interact between the realms of consciousness and the unconscious (Carter, 2010).

The analyst's ability to access multiple levels of consciousness is dependent on the psychic interaction between the analytic dyad. Such interactions result in a countertransference response on the part of the analyst that exposes him or her to the patient's unconscious material, leading to a greater understanding of the patient's internal world while simultaneously providing the analyst with information as to what is occurring during treatment (Kaufmann, 1984). Again, we are seeing the analyst taking on the role of Hermes by making what was previously beyond human understanding into something comprehendible (i.e., making the unconscious conscious). Although the patient's past experiences are of importance, being together in the moment with another individual is also of relevance as "the past reveals itself in the present moment so that repetition is involved, while at the same time the present is always unique and moving toward the potentially predictable but unknown future" (Carter, 2010, p. 202). This again brings us back to the point that countertransference is therefore the fusion between the past and present, the conscious with the unconscious, and a connection between fantasy and reality. Instead of looking at countertransference simply as such, Carter (2010) suggests looking at the analyst's use of self within the analytic relationship, looking at the phenomenological description of the experience, images, metaphors, and amplifications that take place within the interactions. By using such an approach, the interaction between analyst and patient remains open to emergent processes instead of being completely dependent on theory and being seen as a creation within an one-person psychology. For instance, Jung's alchemical process is an example that rejects the one-person approach and, instead, looks at the intra- and inter-psychic aspects of the therapeutic interaction. Carter (2010) states:

> The analyst does not "own" or "have" a countertransference: he is "in" a phenomenological experience co-created with the other. The two people of the analytic dyad are in conjunction, symbolically held by the alchemical vessel constructed through the analytic relationship. . . . Understanding how one is "with another" is essential, along with the capacity for reflective function and for play with metaphor and analogy.
>
> (p. 202)

In other words, as Ogden (1997) stated, the analytic task does not consist of separating the psychological elements belonging to the analyst and patient, but instead of examining the interplay between the two within the transcendent function. The analyst's experience of the transcendent function provides the analyst with an understanding of the conscious and unconscious experiences of the patient's past and present.

Another aspect of the psychic interaction that takes place within the transcendent function involves the dream world of the therapeutic dyad, in particular, the analyst's countertransference dreams. As previously discussed when defining countertransference as a spectrum at the beginning of this chapter, countertransference dreams also fall within a spectrum of possibilities, with dream content ranging from the analyst's own neurosis to the analyst's full experience of the patient (Pollack-Gomolin, 2002). In more specific terms, countertransference dreams highlight the analyst's anxieties related to working with a patient, in addition to revealing important aspects of treatment the analyst was previously unaware of, either in the form of projective identification of the patient's split of the self or by allowing the analyst the opportunity to play out countertransference reactions previously interfering within treatment. Through the use of the transcendent function, the analyst is able to mediate the conscious and unconscious worlds of the patient, bringing both worlds together (Jung, 1958/1969). The mediation of both worlds within the transcendent function allows for the psychic interaction between the dream worlds of the patient and analyst to take place. The psychic interaction allows the analyst to take in the exchange between the patient and analyst, allowing it to manifest within the analyst's dreams. However, to understand the patient's unconscious world, the analyst must be open to such forms of communication and dialogue on behalf of the patient (Jung, 1931/1970; Kron, 1991).

In addition to the psychological interaction between the patient and the analyst, the transcendent function also provides an arena for the therapeutic dyad to communicate within the physical and somatic realm (Ogden, 1997; Gubb, 2014). According to Jung (1931/1970), patients who experience somatic symptoms are capable of transferring their "demon of sickness" onto the analyst. As Jung stated, "a sufferer can transmit his disease to a healthy person whose powers then subdue the demon – but not without impairing the well-being of the subduer" (p. 72). Although Jung did not mention somatic countertransference by name, it is apparent that he was referring to the somatic response evoked by the patient's transference. Somatic countertransference originates within the physical realm of the patient in the form of somatic symptoms; however, as Jung mentioned, the "sickness" or "infection" is then transferred to the analyst, who can deconstruct the patient's unconscious material (Spiegelman, 1996; Beebe, 2004). This, however, does not mean that somatic countertransference is simply the transferring of the patient's illness onto the analyst. As Gubb (2014) stated,

> [i]t is then clear that while there were aspects of both the patient's pathology and the therapist's personality which had played a role in the developing of the somatic response to the patient, it was the interaction of all the relevant elements of the therapeutic dyad which were required for the somatic countertransference to be produced in the form in which it manifested.
>
> (p. 60)

In other words, somatic countertransference follows the same premise as other countertransference responses in that it is a co-constructed phenomenon.

According to Samuels (1985), somatic countertransference is best described as

> a physical, actual, material, sensual expression in the analyst of something in the patient's inner world . . . an incarnation by the analyst of a part of the patient's psyche . . . a 'clothing' by the analyst of the patient's soul.
>
> (p. 52)

Similar to the alchemy and psychic exchange descriptions mentioned in this chapter and the hermeneutic circle of truth, analysts with a somatic countertransference response will submerge themselves into their patients' unconscious material and uses their body as a conduit of sorts to amplify their patients' attempt to communicate with the analysts within the somatic realm. It is important to remember that many countertransference states are nonverbal or pre-verbal, meaning that "the analyst's body is not entirely his or her own and what it says to him or her is not a message from him or her alone" (Samuels, 1989, p. 164). As a result, analysts are expected to work with somatic countertransference responses as they would any other countertransference response. However, somatic countertransference potentially requires additional work due to its manifestation occurring within the somatic versus the psychological realm. The analyst must metabolize the experience in order to bridge the somatic with the psychological, leading to the translation of the somatic response into language and thought (Gubb, 2014).

In order to metabolize and translate the somatic response, Ogden (1997) suggested the use of reverie, allowing the analyst to make meaning of and put into thoughts and words what the patient projected onto the analyst. Gubb (2014), however, warned against the somatic response that becomes noticeable to the patient prior to the analyst. Under certain situations, Gubb (2014) suggested:

> The therapist should be vigilant for such events so that if they bring new material to light when the patient notices the physical response this can be worked with and made use of. When the as yet unprocessed material of the therapist is brought into the room, it is incumbent on the therapist to make use of all the tools available (particularly that of reverie) in order to reveal the meaning of such a response as deeply and thoroughly as possible to themselves first, and then to apply that understanding to that particular therapy's dynamics. These situations may add pressure on the therapist to maintain their analytic stance and not engage in an enactment, but even if slips in these areas do occur, thoughtful and careful analytic work can reveal those underlying dynamics which crave interpretation.
>
> (p. 57)

In other words, through the use of reverie, the analyst is able to metabolize the patient's projection and interpret the relationship between his or her physical response and the patient. The analyst is able to metabolize and mentalize physical symptoms by taking into consideration the moment in which the somatic response took place and attempting to link it to the material the patient brought into session. In the event that the patient notices the somatic response prior to the analyst, ultimately leading to an enactment, it is important for the analyst to work through the enactment by examining his or her own somatic sensations and visuals associated with the enactment and interpret them in relation to the patient's projection. This falls in line with the belief that an analyst does not become aware of their countertransference response until he or she experiences an enactment (Renik, 1993; Devereux, 2006). Enactments, in combination with reverie, provide the analyst with a deeper understanding of the unconscious content, bringing the content into consciousness and the therapeutic space for interpreting and processing.

Returning to the psychological realm of countertransference, the analyst's emotional response and/or reaction to the patient's transference is based on identification with the patient's id, ego, superego, or unconscious representations of the patient's past, and provides the analyst with a view of the patient's internal world (Racker, 1988). The analyst's emotional response assists with the progression of treatment, as it provides the analyst with an avenue in which to identify with the patient's repressed material through the analyst's own thoughts and internal world (Little, 1981; Racker, 1988; Leahy, 2001). For instance, through the use of countertransference, the analyst is able to make interpretations from an emotional standpoint based on the emotions activated by the patient within treatment. As a result, the analyst will experience a spontaneous thought associated with the patient's unconscious. In other words, the analyst becomes a reflection of the patient with the emotional response being a representation of the patient's unconscious, providing the analyst with a direct path into the patient's unconscious and an understanding of their internal world (Heimann, 1950). Countertransference is therefore a requirement for treatment, as it assists in the interpretation and understanding of the patient's transference by providing a portal into the patient's unconscious (Sedgwick, 1994).

Although countertransference responses are directly related to the patient's transference, countertransference manifestations vary in causation and presentation and are directly or indirectly related to the patient (Racker, 1988). For instance, direct countertransference responses come about as a result of the analyst's identification with the patient in one form or another. In one instance, the analyst is able to identify with the patient through an empathic response related to the patient's thoughts and feelings based on projection and introjection. As a result, the analyst is able to feel and identify with the patient while also experiencing the patient's experience through their ability to empathize with the patient, allowing the analyst to experience and understand the patient's psychological state of mind while also providing a view into the patient's unconscious and a deeper understanding of the patient's unconscious material (Paulsen, 1956). Little's (1981) understanding of the psychic exchange between the therapeutic dyad provides the reader with a description of the unconscious interaction between the patient and analyst. According to Little (1981), the analytic work is best described as the analyst holding a mirror in front of the patient and the patient doing the same to the analyst, with the mirrors serving as a method of communication between the patient and analyst. As treatment progresses, a clearer image of the patient presents itself in the mirror; however, the same is also expected of the analyst. The analyst's reflection becomes a representation of the patient's unconscious processes as a result of the analyst's identification with the patient. In other words, the analyst's response is a corresponding identification or reflection of the patient's state of mind and/or experience, allowing for the analyst to experience the patient's unconscious emotional state consciously through the re-experiencing of the analyst's past processes as they relate to the patient (Corbett, 1987; Racker, 1988). Reflective countertransference responses are therefore the analyst's identification with the patient as a result of the analyst's personality identifying with the corresponding psychological part of the patient (i.e., the analyst's id with the patient's id, the analyst's ego with the patient's ego, and the analyst's superego with the patient's superego).

Another form of direct countertransference is initiated by projections on the part of the patient, as opposed to the analyst identifying with the corresponding psychological part of the patient (Racker, 1988). Similar to the Kleinian notion of projective identification, projections on the part of the patient serve as a defense mechanism by the patient's ego and involve the splitting and projection of an unwanted portion of themselves onto the analyst. As a result of the split, the patient is able to reject a toxic introject, or unwanted portion of the ego and/or superego, by identifying the unwanted trait within the analyst. As a result, the patient begins to treat the analyst as an unconscious representation from the past while also identifying the analyst as an individual of past persecution, leading to the analyst's ego identifying with the patient's projection. This identification on the part of the analyst allows for the analyst to experience the patient's projected feelings and impulses toward the patient. Due to the negative transference on the patient's behalf, the analyst experiences a negative countertransference response as a result of the analyst identifying with the patient's persecuting material, leading to the re-projection of the patient's projection. This, however, is not limited to the re-projection of the patient's projection but also the projection of the analyst's own persecutory experiences activated by the patient's projection, leading to a response indirectly related to the patient. In the ideal situation, the analyst is able to accept and tolerate the patient's projection, allowing for the reenactment of the patient's past to take place within the therapeutic setting (Heimann, 1950). Although the analyst accepts and experiences the patient's projections in the same manner as others in the patient's life, the analyst provides the patient with a safe environment to address and explore personal complexes and persecutory experiences, allowing for a reparative experience based on reality to take place. However, when the opposite takes place, the patient becomes a representation of the analyst's past experience, resulting in the analyst feeling threatened by the analysts' superego or unconscious representation of their past. In cases where the analyst acts on his or her own anxieties, the patient re-experiences a reality based on his or her internal world, and is centered on both fantasy and reality. By re-living the experience as a result of the analyst's persecutory countertransference response, the patient's inadequacies are reinforced and the neurosis remains whole instead of being metabolized.

Reflective and persecutory countertransference manifestations are interconnected, requiring the analyst to be completely aware of personal identifications with the patient. For example, by rejecting a part of his or herself, the analyst also rejects a part of the patient, resulting in a persecutory identification with the patient's unconscious representation of their past. If the analyst identifies with the persecutory experience, the analyst reinforces the cause of the patient's neurosis while also hindering progress within treatment. If the analyst does the opposite and accepts their identification with the patient, the analyst becomes an emotional container for the patient, allowing the analyst to interpret and/or analyze their identification and countertransference response while also linking the unconscious response of the analyst with the patient. The linking of unconscious processes provides the analyst with an understanding of what the projected experience invoked within them, enabling the analyst to use that experience as a way of interpreting the patient's transference. Once the patient's projection moves into consciousness, the patient becomes aware of the fact that their present reality does not match their internal perception. As a result, the patient introjects a perception based on reality versus fantasy.

Pathological Countertransference

Although the perception and understanding of countertransference have significantly changed since its introduction by Freud in 1910, many early writings on the phenomenon laid the foundation for understanding the analyst's pathological response, including their origins and interfering nature to treatment. Pathological countertransference responses arise as a result of the analyst's unconscious conflicts-based reaction to the patient's transference (Freud, 1910/1953; Reich, 1951/1990; Klein, 1957/1984; Little, 1981; Winnicott, 1994). The analyst's neurosis, or unresolved conflicts, is a creation of the unconscious part of the analyst's ego by way of the id, and presents themselves in the form of projection and introjection (Little, 1981). Because the analyst's unresolved conflicts are based on early childhood relationships and experiences, the patient becomes a projection of the analyst's past, clouding the analyst's clinical judgment and perception of the patient (Freud, 1910/1953; Reich, 1951/1990). In other words, a phenomenon that recalls the Freud (1912/1953) view of transference and "stereotype plates" that develop based on past experiences also occurs within countertransference, leading to a distorted view of the patient while also interfering with the analyst's ability to distinguish between the patient's past and their own (Gelso & Hayes, 2007). As a result of the analyst's neurosis, pathological countertransference becomes a barrier to the psychological advancement of the patient due to the analyst re-experiencing their neurosis and unresolved conflicts within sessions. Under such circumstances, the analyst will attempt to satisfy their libidinal needs associated with their past, resulting in inaccurate interpretations regarding the patient, leading to the exploitation and manipulation of the patient for the personal gain of the analyst (Little, 1981). In addition, the analyst will over-identify with the patient's experience and re-experience an event from their past, influencing not only their behavior toward the patient but also treatment as a whole (Racker, 1988). Although the analyst's conscious goal of treatment remains focused on the psychological growth of the patient, the analyst unconsciously makes the patient dependent on them by exacerbating an underlying unresolved area. In other words, pathological countertransference prevents the psychological growth of the patient by influencing the unconscious material associated with the primitive needs of the patient's id, hindering the development of the self within the patient (Freud, 1933/1964). Pathological countertransference is therefore a platform for the analyst to act out and alleviate feelings of anxiety and guilt associated with their past experiences.

In theory, difficulties associated with countertransference are commonly related to difficulties with the analysis and interpretation of the patient's transference. As a result, one important aspect to consider when examining the analyst's pathological response is to determine the ego involvement and resulting emotional intensity on the part of the analyst. According to Racker (1988), a low intensity response based on fantasy results from an analogous situation between the analyst and patient, and allows the analyst to understand and communicate with the inner world of the patient. In contrast, a high intensity response by the analyst is the result of the patient acting out. This, however, does not eliminate the role of the analyst within the emotional experience. The analyst can respond either by perceiving and containing their emotional response or by acting out. The analyst's response is dependent on a number of different factors such as their own neurosis, defense mechanisms, and tendency of re-experiencing versus bringing it into consciousness. Under such circumstances, the analyst has one of two options: either they attempt to change their external environment (alloplastic adaption) or they attempt to change their internal world and perceptions (autoplastic adaption). The intensity related to the analyst's countertransference response is, in other words, a defense toward the remembering or reenactment of early childhood experiences and internal conflicts. Such negative countertransference responses are neurotic responses associated with the analyst's unresolved internal conflicts. Although such countertransference responses are inevitable, they still serve a function within treatment. Negative countertransference reactions are a response to the patient's transference neurosis and are not necessarily a bad thing, as they provide the analyst with a view of the patient's internal world. It is important to remember that "in the doctor, his inner wounded side, his own unresolved illnesses, psychic, somatic or both are activated by his contact with the sick person" (Groesbeck, 1975, p. 128). In other words, the analyst's countertransference response serves as a bridge between the internal world of the analyst and patient, bringing to the forefront of treatment the patient's unconscious while also providing the analyst with an understanding of the patient's internal state and underlying difficulties. Of caution to the analyst is the possibility that such a response could also trigger a similar response within the analyst, a response associated with the analyst's neurosis, resulting in the repression of the analyst's countertransference experience by way of the ego and superego. If the response/experience is repressed as a result of their narcissistic wound, the analyst loses the opportunity of gaining a deeper understanding of the patient's transference and internal world. In the event the analyst represses their countertransference response, the patient will attempt to compensate the analyst for not being available due to their perceived ego inferiority as a result of their internal perception of the world. In addition, the patient will use the analyst as a way of seeking equality with an individual of past persecution. As Racker (1988) points out, there are aggressions in the patient's behavior toward the internal representation of a person once perceived as rejecting and superior. By accepting and embracing their countertransference response, the analyst serves the function of the patient's superego, or ego ideal, while simultaneously making the patient aware of their countertransference experience as their response is related to the analyst identifying with the patient's internal representation. By refusing to embrace their countertransference response, the analyst is also rejecting their identification with the patient's internal representation, resulting in the patient re-experiencing the individual of past persecution. To paraphrase Racker (1988), by accepting their deeply emotionally charged responses toward the patient, the analyst serves as a tour guide of sorts, by making the patient aware of their own repressed internal representation and their relationship to them. In other words, the analyst uses their countertransference experience as a way of interpreting the patient's internal word. Through such interpretations, the analyst is able to interrupt the patient's neurosis and re-living their previous experience. In addition, the patient begins to develop a new perception of the individual currently being experienced in the transference, introjecting a reality differing from their internal perceptions.

Although pathological countertransference responses may hinder the forward movement of treatment, not all pathological and/or negative countertransference responses are created equal. According to Winnicott (1994), countertransference develops as a result of the psychological burden placed on the analyst, resulting in the development of negative feelings toward the patient. Such responses are important to be aware of as they provide the analyst with a view into the patient's behaviors and personality via the emotional response of the analyst. In other words, negative countertransference responses provide the analyst with a reflection or firsthand experience of how the patient makes others feel and what reactions others experience as a result of the patient; hence, interpreting the analyst's emotional response to the patient provides the analyst with an understanding of the reactions others experience through their interactions with the patient (Racker, 1988; Leahy, 2001; Gelso & Hayes, 2007).

Distance

Although it remains difficult to differentiate between pathological and non-pathological countertransference responses, the analyst is encouraged to accept their countertransference response while at the same time distancing themselves from the patient's experience. If the analyst accepts their countertransference response, they are able to decipher the material that needs to be interpreted within treatment, while also exploring their own emotional response toward the patient (Racker, 1988). Rejecting their response not only leads to a pathological response on the part of the analyst but also leads to the rejection of a part of the patient. As a way of preventing a pathological response, Little (1981) encouraged the distancing or detachment of the analyst from the patient's experience, however, not in the same frame of mind as Freud. Instead of the Freudian belief related to the detached surgeon, Little encouraged empathizing and identifying with the patient while remaining detached from the patient's experience. In other words, the analyst is expected to "discover how to be psychologically intimate with a patient yet separate, separate and still intimate" (Casement,

1985, p. 30). If the analyst experiences a presentness to the patient's experience and is unable to separate themselves as a result of the ego's inability to detach, the analyst will take ownership of the patient's experience. If the analyst has gone through a similar experience, the ego is able to detach from the experience as a result of the time that has elapsed between the analyst and their experience, allowing for the immediacy between the patient and the experience. According to Gadamer's concept of historical consciousness, the same element that provides the distancing from a patient's experience is also what connects us to their past experiences: time (Gadamer, 2004). As Zimmermann (2015) stated,

> history is like a stream in which we move and participate in every act of understanding. The very reason that we can understand anything at all from the past is because we already stand in a stream of time that connects past and present.
>
> (p. 41)

In other words, the analyst is familiar with the experience as it relates to their past while the patient is familiar with the experience as a result of it being their present, making the experience solely that of the patient, automatically introducing the element of distance to the experience. In order for countertransference to be effective, the elements of time and distance must be present, allowing for the introjective identification of the patient. Distance and time are therefore critical elements within countertransference as they promote growth while also prompting identification and separation for the analyst.

Analysis of the Analyst

According to Jung (1937/1970), the treatment of patients is an ongoing stress-provoking occurrence, making the analyst susceptible to countertransference reactions resulting from personal complexes and unmet libidinal needs, leading to the stagnation of treatment. The analyst's susceptibility to countertransference, however, is not necessarily related to their neurosis alone but also to the extensiveness of the analyst's unconsciousness, an unconscious realm co-created in conjunction with the patient. As Jung (1931/1970) argued, the analyst "is equally part of the psychic process of treatment and therefore equally exposed to the transforming influences. Indeed, to the extent that the doctor shows himself impervious to this influence, he forfeits influence over the patient" (p. 72). As a result of the shared unconscious space and potential reactions resulting from it, countertransference is seen as a "psychic infection" or a potential sickness transferred from the patient to the analyst by way of their shared unconsciousness (Jung, 1931/1970). Winnicott (1994) also warned against the derailment of treatment resulting from the "psychological burden" placed on the analyst via their countertransference responses. Given that countertransference is a co-constructed phenomenon that involves a mutual transformation for those involved, Jung argued that "the stronger and more stable personality" will have a stronger pull on the other (p. 72). To prevent derailments related to such infections or psychological burdens, analysts are highly encouraged to enter their own analysis as a way of uncovering their personal blind spots and/or to rid themselves of residual pathology related to past conflicts and experiences (Freud, 1912/1953; Jung, 1931/1970; Heimann, 1950; Klein, 1957/1984; Little, 1981; Racker, 1988; Winnicott, 1994; Leahy, 2001; Prasko et al., 2010). As Samuels (1985) stated,

> [i]t should be added that not all countertransference reactions are usable communications from the patient. We need to bare neurotic countertrans-ference in mind – identifying with the patient, idealising the patient, the analyst's relation to the patient's aggression, his destruction of his own work, his attempt to satisfy his own infantile needs through his relation-ship with the patient. Nor is it always immediately clear what the patient's communications mean. As Jung stated, the analyst may have to stay in a muddled, bewildered state for a period, allowing his understanding to germinate, if it will. His ability to rest with his anxiety and maintain his attitude of affective involvement becomes crucial.
>
> (pp. 53–54)

Clark (2006) and Merchant (2012) also stressed the need for the analyst to be aware of their personal vulnerabilities as a result of countertransferential infor-mation, in particular, psychic and somatic responses, being received through the analyst's weakest or most problematic areas. As a way of preventing the potential of a psychic infection, the analyst's own analysis allows the analyst to develop a relationship with their own complexes, leading the analyst to use their personal experiences as a source of trusted information (Merchant, 2012). Although the patient and analyst encountered different experiences, the ana-lyst's vulnerabilities have the potential of becoming reactive to the patient's material, once again stressing the need for the analysis of the analyst. As Case-ment (1985) explained, "the patient needs to be allowed opportunities for opti-mum experiences, without interference from the therapist" (p. 29). However, if the analyst is resistant to their own analysis, their personal conflicts and unmet libidinal needs will interfere with treatment and the analyst will encounter dif-ficulties associated with the patient's transference.

According to Heimann (1950), pathological and nonpathological counter-transference responses are commonly mishandled, resulting in poor interpreta-tions on the part of the analyst. In theory, if the analyst goes through their own analysis, the analyst is able to address their personal conflicts and neurosis, leading to their emotional stability. If emotionally stable, the analyst develops the ability to follow the emotional responses and unconscious material of the patient in conjunction with the patient's associations and how they relate to the analyst's emotional response. However, if the analyst has not addressed their own conflicts and neurosis and they lack emotional stability, they will proj-ect what rightfully belongs to them onto the patient, resulting in problematic interpretations of the patient's transference. This, in turn, brings us back to Little's mirror analogy (Little, 1981). If the analyst is resistant to exploring and addressing their conflicts and neurosis, the mirror providing their reflection will remain hazed or re-hazed as a result of their resistance. In addition, the hazing or re-hazing of the mirror interferes with the analyst's ability to distance themselves from the patient's experience, leading to the analyst claiming the patient's experience as their own. The analyst's inability to distance themselves from the patient's experience in turn leads to a distancing between the patient and analyst. If the patient experiences a distancing from the analyst, the patient will attempt to break down the analyst's resistance as a way of connecting with the analyst while also introjecting their experience of the analyst, a reality-based experience that reinforces the patient's neurosis, and ultimately leads to a greater resistance within the patient.

In the ideal situation, the analyst is able to accept and tolerate the patient's projections, leading to the reenactment of experiences from the patient's past within the therapeutic relationship. However, if the analyst is resistant to their own analysis, they will project their own unresolved conflicts onto the patient. For example, under such circumstances, the patient will activate an unresolved issue within the analyst (i.e., the patient reveals being unfaithful in their relationship) and the analyst will project that onto the patient (i.e., the analyst begins feeling a sense of dislike toward the patient as a result of their significant other being unfaithful toward them). As a result, Heimann (1950) stressed the importance of the analyst's acknowledging and mastering unresolved conflicts to prevent the projection of issues onto the patient. This, however, does not suggest the need to eliminate the analyst's emotional or countertransference response toward the patient. Instead, through the use of their countertransference responses, the analyst is able to gain an understanding of the patient's unconscious and reflect that to the patient in the form of interpretations. The emotions experienced by the analyst are useful therapeutic tools, as they provide insight into the patient's unconscious conflicts and defenses. As a result, changes within the patient's ego occur as well as the strengthening of the patient's sense of reality, ultimately allowing the patient to see the analyst as simply another person and not an individual to idealize. By undergoing personal analysis, the analyst is able to deal with personal issues and by extension is able to assist the patient on how to deal with his or her own personal difficulties (Jung, 1931/1970). The analyst's need for personal analysis leads to a circular system which allows the analyst to learn continually about themselves as patients awaken unconscious material previously hibernating within the analyst. When looking at countertransference, it is important to consider the description Villard (2013) gave when discussing the anticipated Milky Way/Andromeda collision: "A baseball batter knows that a pitched ball is coming toward him, but he has to decide whether it will be over the middle of the plate, a bit inside, or at his head" (p. 25). Analysts are required to make a similar decision about deciding whether to seek or resist their own analysis. Resisting their own analysis can cause treatment to go stagnant, as patients are unable to progress within treatment as a result of analysts' inability to deal with their own neurosis. The analysis of the analyst provides the analyst with an opportunity to explore and address their own complexes and neuroses. Eliot (1932) wrote,

> [a]nd he is not likely to know what is to be done unless he lives in what is not merely the present, but the present moment of the past, unless he is conscious, not of what is dead, but of what is already living.
>
> (p. 11)

In other words, by going through their own analysis, the analyst is able to embrace his or her own woundedness, which in turn allows the analyst to understand the woundedness of others. In addition, by having a greater understanding of his or her own psychological wounds, the analyst develops a greater sense of empathy toward the patient. As Jung (1989) stated, "the doctor is effective only when he himself is affected" (p. 134). In other words, the ability to understand others is closely connected with analysts' ability to understand themselves.

8   Moving Forward
Implications and Recommendations

The intent of this inquiry has been to probe and understand the analyst's intersubjective experience and the role it plays within the therapeutic setting. Although a number of writings currently exist that focus on the analyst's intersubjective experience, writings are theory specific and have led to an overall absence of a standard and universal definition of the phenomenon. By engaging in a hermeneutic dialogue with a number of theoretical writings focused on the phenomenon of countertransference, the researcher was able to embody the messenger-god Hermes by bridging the past with the present, and the old with the new. Such an approach led to the creation of a more comprehensive level of understanding, and ultimately, a transtheoretical definition of countertransference. This concluding chapter will focus on the benefits of a transtheoretical definition of countertransference to the field of psychology and its applications to the field. In addition, this chapter concludes with recommendations for future research and methodological considerations.

Benefits and Applications to the Field

Traditionally, the concept of countertransference is based on psychodynamic tenets; however, experiencing a subjective experience with patient material is unavoidable and an intricate part of psychotherapy regardless of theoretical orientation. While engaging in a hermeneutic dialogue with the selected texts, the researcher encountered a pleasant but unexpected surprise: many theoretical approaches address countertransference; however, each theoretical frame of mind uses theory-specific language. In other words, the field of psychology has attempted to conceptualize the phenomenon of countertransference in a manner equivalent to having a number of individuals who all speak different languages trying to communicate with each other, making it nearly impossible. By developing a transtheoretical understanding of countertransference, the researcher served as an interpreter of sorts, providing analysts with a generic language that allows them to communicate and understand each other to their fullest capacity. Similar to Jon Kabat-Zinn's approach while developing his Mindfulness-Based Stress Reduction treatment (Husgafvel, 2016), the researcher developed a generic language that allows for a universal understanding of

DOI: 10.4324/9781003320180-9

countertransference while also removing the phenomenon from psychodynamic theory. Returning to the Mindfulness-Based Stress Reduction example, Kabat-Zinn implemented the practice of Buddhist meditation as a form of treatment for chronic pain and stress reduction, although he removed it from Buddhist and religious practices (Husgafvel, 2016). According to Kabat-Zinn,

> [w]hile the most systematic and comprehensive articulation of mindfulness and its related attributes stems from the Buddhist tradition, mindfulness is not a catechism, an ideology, a belief system, a technique or set of techniques, a religion, or a philosophy. It is best described as "a way of being".
> (as cited in Husgafvel, 2016, p. 88)

By removing the practice from Buddhist traditions and instead describing it as "a way of being," Mindfulness-Based Stress Reduction became widely accepted and is commonly used in the treatment of a variety of psychiatric conditions (Goldberg, Knoeppel, Davidson, & Flook, 2020). In using a similar approach, the hope is that individuals working from a non-depth psychological approach will ultimately gain not only a more comprehensive understanding of the phenomenon of countertransference but also an acceptance and understanding of how to integrate the use of countertransference within treatment.

A transtheoretical approach to countertransference also promotes the clinical growth of the analyst as the analyst develops the ability of identifying the different forms of countertransference, and deciphering between the beneficial forms of countertransference and those interfering with treatment. By extension, understanding the interfering aspects of countertransference leads to the personal growth of the analyst as the analyst develops an understanding of their global response to the patient through their personal experience of the patient and the analytic setting. Understanding their countertransference response requires a vulnerability and willingness on the part of the analyst to know themselves in order to determine if their response is associated with the patient or their own unresolved unconscious conflicts. If the analyst is used as a channel for translating and understanding the patient's unconscious material as a way of bringing it into consciousness, the path from the unconscious to consciousness requires the clearest road possible to ensure proper interpretations on the part of the analyst. In other words, the clinical and personal growth of the analyst brought on by a more comprehensive understanding of countertransference ultimately leads to a greater understanding and acceptance of the patient and the analyst themselves.

Limitations and Recommendations for Future Research

Although a robust sample of theoretical writings was selected for interpretation during this philosophical hermeneutic inquiry, not all theoretical perspectives were included. Influential minds such as those of Alfred Adler, Wilfred Bion, James Hillman, and Marie-Louise von Franz, to name a few, were not included in this study. In addition, philosophical hermeneutic inquiries are categorized as qualitative research and therefore do not meet the standard of evidence-based research. This, however, does not render this inquiry useless. Unlike quantitative research that focuses on cause and effect and treatment effectiveness from a statistical standpoint, qualitative research focuses on the personal experience of others by telling their story, an aspect of research that quantitative approaches are incapable of measuring. Future research should focus on expanding the foundation of this inquiry by including additional theoretical writings and approaches to countertransference. This expansion would also include the further development of a neutral language model that encompasses the benefits and challenges associated with countertransference as a way of adapting it to non-psychodynamic practices. In addition, conducting a quantitative study involving analysts/therapists practicing from a wide range of theoretical approaches that focuses on their subjective experiences with their patients, and their perception of benefits and hindrances related to countertransference would further assist in identifying the gaps remaining between depth psychological approaches to countertransference and those of non-psychodynamic practices. Identifying such gaps provides future researchers with insight into the areas of countertransference that still need to be addressed and generalized.

Conclusion

Over the past century, the meaning and understanding of countertransference have continuously evolved, an evolution that continues today. Although the meaning and understanding of countertransference remain fluid, a universal understanding of the phenomenon understood across theoretical orientations continued to elude the field of psychology. Most definitions of countertransference remain theory specific and are explained using theory-specific language, in particular, that of depth psychological approaches. As a result, the therapeutic use of countertransference remains an underutilized skill, even though countertransference remains an ever present occurrence in treatment across theoretical approaches. In theory, it is difficult to implement a skill that one has not been trained in or that one does not understand. The purpose of this philosophical hermeneutic inquiry aimed to change that by bridging the gaps between theoretical approaches and developing a transtheoretical understanding of countertransference. In addition, while interpreting the text, one conclusion became evident: the evolution of countertransference appeared to be linked with the evolution of the writers as individuals and their willingness to know themselves, a point of inquiry that presented itself in the research. Unlike the initial Freudian view on countertransference that encouraged the analyst to avoid any emotional response to the patient, as it could symbolize the unmet libidinal needs of the analyst, more recent writings encourage analysts to understand their emotional response as a way of determining its origin and rightful owner. It is important to remember that countertransference is not simply transference on the part of the analyst but a mode of communication between the patient and analyst. Countertransference allows the patient to tell his or her story through the use of the analyst while also allowing the analyst to understand the patient's experience. Countertransference, however, is not the be-all and end-all of treatment but instead is a method of understanding. A transtheoretical approach to countertransference promotes such a level of understanding through the use of the analyst without the need of becoming immersed in psychodynamic theory.

References

Abramovitch, H., & Lange, T. (1994). Dreaming about my patient: A case illustration of the therapist's initial dream. *Dreaming, 4*(2), 105–113.

Adams, M. V. (2008). The archetypal school. In P. Young-Eisendrath & T. Dawson (Eds.), *The Cambridge companion to Jung* (2nd ed., pp. 107–124). New York: Cambridge University Press.

Agnel, A. (1992). Another degree of complexity. In M. A. Matoon (Ed.), *Chicago 92: The transcendent function – Individual and collective aspects: Proceedings of the Twelfth International Congress for Analytical Psychology* (pp. 101–115). Einsiedeln, Switzerland: Daimon Verlag.

Aron, L. (1991). The patient's experience of the analyst's subjectivity. In S. Mitchell & L. Aron (Eds.), *Relational perspectives: The emergence of a tradition* (pp. 245–268). Hillsdale, NJ: The Analytic Press.

Aron, L. (1993). Working toward operational thought: Piagetian theory and psychoanalytic method. *Contemporary Psychoanalysis, 29,* 289–313.

Aron, L. (1996). *A meeting of minds: Mutuality in psychoanalysis.* Hillsdale, NJ: Analytic Press.

Aron, L. (1998). The clinical body and the reflexive mind. In L. Aron & F. S. Anderson (Eds.), *Relational perspectives on the body* (pp. 3–38). Hillsdale, NJ: The Analytic Press.

Bach, S. (1985). *Narcissistic states and the therapeutic process.* New York: Aronson.

Beebe, J. (2004). Understanding consciousness through the theory of psychological types. In J. Cambray & L. Carter (Eds.), *Analytical psychology* (pp. 83–115). New York: Brunner-Routledge.

Bugental, J. (1978). *Psychotherapy and process: The fundamentals of an existential-humanistic approach.* Reading, MA: Addison-Wesley.

Bugental, J. (1987). *The art of the psychotherapist.* New York: Norton.

Carter, L. (2010). Countertransference and intersubjectivity. In M. Stein (Ed.), *Jungian psychoanalysis* (pp. 201–212). Chicago, IL: Open Court Press.

Casement, P. J. (1985). *On learning from the patient.* New York: Guilford Press.

Clark, G. (2006). A Spinozan lens onto the confusions of borderline relations. *Journal of Analytical Psychology, 51,* 67–86.

Corbett, L. (1987). Psychology of the transference and countertransference. Talk presented at *1987 C. G. Jung Institute of Chicago,* Evanston, IL.

Corsini, R. J. (2016). *The dictionary of psychology.* New York: Routledge.

Cox, T. J., & Loeb, A. (2008). The collision between the Milky Way and Andromeda. *Monthly Notices of the Royal Astronomical Society, 386*(1), 461–474.

Curtis, J. M. (1981). Indications and contra-indications in the use of therapist's self-disclosure. *Psychology Reports, 49*, 499–507.

Cvetovac, M. E., & Adame, A. L. (2017). The wounded therapist: Understanding the relationship between personal suffering and clinical practice. *The Humanistic Psychologist, 45*(4), 348–366.

Devereux, D. (2006). Enactment: Some thoughts about the therapist's contribution. *British Journal of Psychotherapy, 22*(4), 497–508.

Diffin, A. (2019). *The psychic exchange* [Digital]. Long Beach, CA.

Eliot, T. (1932). *Selected essays: 1917–1932*. New York: Harcourt.

Ellis, A. (2001). Rational and irrational aspects of countertransference. *Journal of Clinical Psychology, 57*, 999–1004.

Epstein, L., & Feiner, A. H. (1988). Countertransference: The therapist's contribution to treatment. In B. Wolstein (Ed.), *Essential papers on countertransference* (pp. 282–303). New York: University Press.

Favero, M., & Ross, D. R. (2002). Complementary dreams: A window to the subconscious processes of countertransference and subjectivity. *American Journal of Psychotherapy, 56*(2), 211–224.

Ferenczi, S., & Rank, O. (1923). The development of psychoanalysis. *Journal of the American Psychoanalytic Association, 42*(3), 851–862.

Fodor, N., & Gaynor, F. (Eds.). (1966). *Freud: Dictionary of psychoanalysis*. Greenwich, CT: Fawcett.

Freud, S. (1953). The future prospects of psycho-analytic therapy. In J. Riviere (Trans.), *The collected papers of Sigmund Freud, Vol. II* (pp. 285–296). London: Hogarth Press (Original work published 1910).

Freud, S. (1953). Recommendations for physicians on the psycho-analytic method of treatment. In J. Riviere (Trans.), *The collected papers of Sigmund Freud, Vol. II* (pp. 323–333). London: Hogarth Press (Original work published 1912).

Freud, S. (1953). Turnings in the ways of psycho-analytic therapy. In J. Riviere (Trans.), *The collected papers of Sigmund Freud, Vol. II* (pp. 392–402). London: Hogarth Press (Original work published 1919).

Freud, S. (1958). The dynamics of transference. In J. Strachey (Ed. & Trans.), *The standard edition of the complete psychological works of Sigmund Freud, Vol. 12* (pp. 97–108). London: Hogarth Press (Original work published 1912).

Freud, S. (1958). Remembering, repeating, and working through (Further recommendations on the technique of psycho-analysis II). In J. Strachey (Ed. & Trans.), *The standard edition of the complete psychological works of Sigmund Freud, Vol. 12* (pp. 145–156). London: Hogarth Press (Original work published 1914).

Freud, S. (1958). Observations on transference-love (Further recommendations on the technique of psycho-analysis III). In J. Strachey (Ed. & Trans.), *The standard edition of the complete psychological works of Sigmund Freud, Vol. 12* (pp. 157–171). London: Hogarth Press (Original work published 1915).

Freud, S. (1963). General theory of the neurosis. In J. Strachey (Ed. & Trans.), *The standard edition of the complete psychological works of Sigmund Freud, Vol. 16* (pp. 243–463). London: Hogarth Press (Original work published 1917).

Freud, S. (1964). Fragment of an analysis of a case of hysteria. In J. Strachey (Ed. & Trans.), *The standard edition of the complete psychological works of Sigmund Freud, Vol. 7* (pp. 7–122). London: Hogarth Press (Original work published 1905).

Freud, S. (1964). New introductory lectures on psycho-analysis. In J. Strachey (Ed. & Trans.), *The standard edition of the complete psychological works of Sigmund Freud, Vol. 22* (pp. 7–182). London: Hogarth Press (Original work published 1933).

Freud, S. (1966). *The basic writings of Sigmund Freud* (A. A. Brill, Ed. & Trans.). New York: Modern Library.

Gadamer, H. (2004). *Truth and method* (2nd, rev. ed.) (J. Weinsheimer & D. G. Marshall Trans.). New York: Continuum (Original work published 1975).

Gelso, C. J., & Hayes, J. A. (2007). *Countertransference and the therapist's inner experience: Perils and possibilities*. Mahwah, NJ: Erlbaum.

Gieser, S. (2005). *The innermost kernel: Depth psychology and quantum physics. Wolfgang Pauli's dialogue with C. G. Jung*. Berlin, Germany: Springer.

Gitelson, M. (1952). The emotional position of the analyst in the psycho-analytic situation. *International Journal of Psychoanalysis, 33*, 1–10.

Glover, E. (1924). Lectures on technique in psycho-analysis. *International Journal of Psychoanalysis, 8*, 311–338; 486–520.

Goldberg, S. B., Knoeppel, C., Davidson, R. J., & Flook, L. (2020). Does practice quality mediate the relationship between practice time and outcome in mindfulness-based stress reduction? *Journal of Counseling Psychology, 67*(1), 115–122. https://doi-org.pgi.idm.oclc.org/10.1037/cou0000369.supp (Supplemental)

Goldfried, M. R., & Davison, G. C. (1994). *Clinical behavior therapy*. New York: Wiley.

Gordon, R. M., Gazzillo, F., Blake, A., Bornstein, R. F., Etzi, J., Lingiardi, V., McWilliams, N., Rothery, C., & Tasso, A. F. (2016). The relationship between theoretical orientation and countertransference expectations: Implications for ethical dilemmas and risk management. *Clinical Psychology and Psychotherapy, 23*(3), 236–245.

Greenberg, J. R., & Mitchell, S. A. (1983). *Object relations in psychoanalytic theory*. Cambridge, MA: Harvard University Press.

Groesbeck, C. J. (1975). The archetypal image of the wounded healer. *Journal of Analytical Psychology, 20*(2), 122–145.

Gubb, K. (2014). Craving interpretation: A case of somatic countertransference. *British Journal of Psychotherapy, 30*(1), 51–67.

Habibi-Kohlen, D. (2018). Paths of the countertransference in the analyst – Clinical examples of working through. *The International Journal of Psychoanalysis, 99*(2), 391–410.

Heimann, P. (1950). On counter-transference. *International Journal of Psycho-Analysis, 31*, 81–84. Retrieved from https://search-ebscohost-com.pgi.idm.oclc.org/login.aspx?direct=true&db=pph&AN=IJP.031.0081A&site=ehost-live&scope=site

Husgafvel, V. (2016). On the Buddhist roots of contemporary non-religious mindfulness practice: Moving beyond sectarian and essentialist approaches. *Temenos, 52*(1), 87–126.

Jacoby, M. (1984). *The analytic encounter: Transference and human relationship*. Toronto, Canada: Inner City Books.

Jung, C. G. (1964). Role of the unconscious. In R. F. C. Hull (Trans.), *The collected works of C. G. Jung, Vol. 10: Civilization in transition* (pp. 3–28). New York: Bollingen (Original work published 1918).

Jung, C. G. (1968a). *Analytical psychology: Its theory and practice (The Tavistock lectures)*. New York: Pantheon Books.

Jung, C. G. (1968b). *The collected works of C. G. Jung, Vol. 12: Psychology and alchemy* (2nd ed.) (R. F. C. Hull, Trans.). Princeton, NJ: Princeton University Press.

Jung, C. G. (1969). General aspects of dream psychology. In R. F. C. Hull (Trans.), *The collected works of C. G. Jung, Vol. 8: The structure and dynamics of the psyche*

(2nd ed., pp. 237–280). Princeton, NJ: Princeton University Press (Original work published 1948).

Jung, C. G. (1969). Archetypes of the collective unconscious. In R. F. C. Hull (Trans.), *The collected works of C. G. Jung, Vol. 9, Part 1: The archetypes and the collective unconscious* (2nd ed., pp. 3–41). Princeton, NJ: Princeton University Press (Original work published 1954).

Jung, C. G. (1969). The transcendent function. In R. F. C. Hull (Trans.), *The collected works of C. G. Jung, Vol. 8: The structure and dynamics of the psyche* (2nd ed., pp. 67–91). Princeton, NJ: Princeton University Press (Original work published 1958).

Jung, C. G. (1970). Problems of modern psychotherapy. In R. F. C. Hull (Trans.), *The collected works of C. G. Jung, Vol. 16: The practice of psychotherapy* (2nd ed., pp. 53–75). Princeton, NJ: Princeton University Press (Original work published 1931).

Jung, C. G. (1970). Principles of practical psychotherapy. In R. F. C. Hull (Trans.), *The collected works of C. G. Jung, Vol. 16: The practice of psychotherapy* (2nd ed., pp. 3–20). Princeton, NJ: Princeton University Press (Original work published 1935).

Jung, C. G. (1970). The realities of practical psychotherapy. In R. F. C. Hull (Trans.), *The collected works of C. G. Jung, Vol. 16: The practice of psychotherapy* (2nd ed., pp. 327–338). Princeton, NJ: Princeton University Press (Original work published 1937).

Jung, C. G. (1970). The psychology of the transference. In R. F. C. Hull (Trans.), *The collected works of C. G. Jung, Vol. 16: The practice of psychotherapy* (2nd ed., pp. 163–323). Princeton, NJ: Princeton University Press (Original work published 1946).

Jung, C. G. (1970). Fundamental questions of psychotherapy. In R. F. C. Hull (Trans.), *The collected works of C. G. Jung, Vol. 16: The practice of psychotherapy* (2nd ed., pp. 111–125). Princeton, NJ: Princeton University Press (Original work published 1951).

Jung, C. G. (1971). *The collected works of C. G. Jung, Vol. 6: Psychological types* (R. F. C. Hull (Trans.). Princeton, NJ: Princeton University Press.

Jung, C. G. (1989). *Memories, dreams, reflections* (A. Jaffe, Ed.). New York: Vintage Books.

Kafle, N. P. (2011). Hermeneutic phenomenological research method simplified. *Bodhi: An Interdisciplinary Journal, 5,* 181–200

Kalsched, D. (1996). *The inner world of trauma.* London: Routledge

Kalsched, D. (2013). *Trauma and the soul.* New York: Routledge.

Karamanolaki, H. (2008). Clinical notes on the inner experiences of the analyst. *International Forum of Psychoanalysis, 17*(1), 44–50.

Kaufmann, Y. (1984). Analytical psychotherapy. In R. J. Corsini (Ed.), *Current psychotherapies* (3rd ed., pp. 108–141). Itasca, IL: Peacock.

Kernberg, O. F. (1992). *Aggression in personality disorders and perversions.* New Haven, CT: Yale University Press.

Klein, M. (1984). Notes on some schizoid mechanisms. In R. Money-Kyrle (Ed.), *The writings of Melanie Klein, Vol. III: Envy and gratitude, and other works* (pp. 1–24). New York: Free Press (Original work published 1946).

Klein, M. (1984). The origins of transference. In R. Money-Kyrle (Ed.), *The writings of Melanie Klein, Vol. III: Envy and gratitude, and other works* (pp. 48–56). New York: Free Press (Original work published 1952).

Klein, M. (1984). Envy and gratitude. In R. Money-Kyrle (Ed.), *The writings of Melanie Klein, Vol. III: Envy and gratitude, and other works* (pp. 176–235). New York: Free Press (Original work published 1957).

Kron, T. (1991). The dialogical dimension in therapists' dreams about their patients. *Israel Journal of Psychiatry and Related Sciences, 28,* 1–12.

Langs, R. (1976). *The therapeutic interaction*. New York: Aronson.

Leahy, R. L. (2001). *Overcoming resistance in cognitive therapy*. New York: Guilford Press.

Lia, M. (2017). Reflections, and relative examples, regarding countertransference, empathy, and observation. *International Forum of Psychoanalysis, 26*(2), 85–96.

Little, M. (1981). *Transference neurosis and transference psychosis*. New York: Aronson.

Machtiger, H. G. (1982). Countertransference/transference. In M. Stein (Ed.), *Jungian analysis* (pp. 88–110). La Salle, IL: Open Court.

Martin, S. (2001). *Alchemy and alchemists*. Chicago, IL: Pocket Essentials.

McClure, B. A., & Hodge, R. W. (1987). Measuring countertransference and attitude in therapists. *American Journal of Psychotherapy, 42*, 521–531.

Meador, B. D., & Rogers, C. R. (1984). Client-centered therapy. In R. J. Corsini (Ed.), *Current psychotherapies* (3rd ed., pp. 142–195). Itasca, IL: Peacock.

Meier, C. A. (1959). Projection, transference, and the subject-object relation in psychology. *Journal of Analytic Psychology, 4*(1), 21–34.

Merchant, J. (2012). *Shamans and analysts: New insights on the wounded healer*. New York: Routledge.

Miller, J. C. (2004). *The transcendent function*. New York: State University of New York Press.

Murdock, N. (2004). *Theories of counseling and psychotherapy: A case approach*. Upper Saddle River, NJ: Pearson.

Myers, W. A. (1987). Work on countertransference facilitated by self-analysis of the analyst's dreams. In A. Rothstein (Ed.), *The interpretation of dreams in clinical work* (pp. 37–46). Madison, CT: International Universities Press.

Natterson, J. (1991). *Beyond countertransference: The therapist's subjectivity in the therapeutic process*. Northvale, NJ: Aronson.

Newman, K. D. (1980). Countertransference and consciousness. *Spring*, 117–127.

Ogden, T. H. (1979). On projective identification. *International Journal of Psychoanalysis, 60*, 371–394.

Ogden, T. H. (1984). Instinct, phantasy, and psychological deep structure: A reinterpretation of aspects of the work of Melanie Klein. *Contemporary Psychoanalysis, 20*, 500–525.

Ogden, T. H. (1997). Reverie and metaphor: Some thoughts on how I work as a psychoanalyst. *International Journal of Psychoanalysis, 78*, 719–732.

Orr, D. (1954). Transference and countertransference: A historical survey. In B. Wolstein (Ed.), *Essential papers on countertransference* (pp. 91–110). New York: New York University Press.

Packer, M., & Addison, R. (1989). *Entering the circle: Hermeneutic investigation in psychology*. Albany, NY: State University of New York Press.

Palmer, R. (1969). *Hermeneutics: Interpretation theory in Schleiermacher, Dilthey, Heidegger and Gadamer*. Evanston, IL: Northwestern University Press.

Park, J. (2018). Sizing up Andromeda. *Astronomy, 46*(6), 19.

Paterson, M., & Higgs, J. (2005). Using hermeneutics as a qualitative research approach in professional practice. *The Qualitative Report, 10*(2), 339–357.

Paulsen, L. (1956). Transference and projection. *Journal of Analytic Psychology, 1*(2), 203–206.

Plaut, A. (1956). The transference in analytical psychology. In M. Fordham (Ed.), *Technique in Jungian analysis* (pp. 152–160). London: Heinemann Medical.

Pollack-Gomolin, R. (2002). The countertransference dream. *Modern Psychoanalysis, 27*(1), 51–75.

Prasko, J., Diveky, T., Grambal, A., Kamaradova, D., Mozny, P., Sigmundova, Z., Slepecky, M., & Vyskocilova, J. (2010). Transference and countertransference in cognitive behavioral therapy. *Biomedical Papers, 154*(3), 189–198.

Racker, H. (1968). *Transference and countertransference.* New York: International Universities Press.

Racker, H. (1988). The meaning and uses of countertransference. In B. Wolstein (Ed.), *Essential papers on countertransference* (pp. 158–201). New York: New York University Press.

Redgrove, H. S. (1997). *Alchemy: Ancient and modern.* Charlottesville, VA: A Mystical World Reprints.

Reich, A. (1960). Further remarks on countertransference. *International Journal of Psycho-Analysis, 41*, 389–395.

Reich, A. (1990). On counter-transference. In R. Langs (Ed.), *Classics in psychoanalytic technique* (pp. 153–160). Lanham, MD: Rowman and Littlefield (Original work published 1951).

Reich, W. (1947). *Character-analysis.* New York: The Noonday Press.

Renik, O. (1993). Analytic interaction: Conceptualizing technique in light of the analyst's irreducible subjectivity. *Psychoanalytic Quarterly, 62*, 553–571.

Renik, O. (1999). Playing one's cards face up in analysis: An approach to the problem of self-disclosure. *Psychoanalytic Quarterly, 62*, 521–539.

Rogers, C. R. (1961). *On becoming a person: A therapist's view of psychotherapy.* Boston, MA: Houghton Mifflin.

Rogers, C. R. (2007). The necessary and sufficient conditions of therapeutic personality change. *Psychotherapy: Theory, Research, Practice, Training, 44*(3), 240–248.

Romanyshyn, R. (2007). *The wounded researcher.* New Orleans, LA: Spring Journal Books.

Rudd, M. D., & Joiner, T. (1997). Countertransference and the therapeutic relationship: A cognitive perspective. *Journal of Cognitive Psychotherapy, 11*, 231–250.

Samuels, A. (1985). Countertransference, the "mundus imaginalis" and a research project. *Journal of Analytical psychology, 30*(1), 47–71.

Samuels, A. (1989). *The plural psyche: Personality, morality and the father.* London: Routledge.

Scharff, J., & Scharff, D. E. (1998). *Object relations individual therapy.* Northvale, NJ: Aronson.

Searles, H. F. (1958). The schizophrenic's vulnerability to the therapist's unconscious processes. In H. F. Searles (Ed.), *Collected papers on schizophrenia and related subjects* (pp. 192–215). New York: International Universities Press.

Sedgwick, D. (1994). *The wounded healer: Countertransference from a Jungian perspective.* Philadelphia, PA: Brunner-Routledge.

Segal, J. (1992). *Melanie Klein.* London: Sage.

Sharp, D. (1991). *C. G. Jung lexicon: A primer of terms and concepts.* Toronto, Canada: Inner City Books.

Spiegelman, J. M. (1996). *Psychotherapy as a mutual process.* Tempe, AZ: New Falcon.

Spillius, E. B. (Ed.). (1988). *Melanie Klein today: Developments in practice, vol. 2: Mainly practice.* New York: Routledge.

Spillius, E. B., Milton, J., Garvey, P., Couve, C., & Steiner, D. (2011). *The new dictionary of Kleinian thought.* New York: Taylor and Francis.

Stern, A. (1924). On the counter-transference in psychoanalysis. *Psychoanalytic Review*, *11*, 166–174.

Stolorow, R. D., & Atwood, G. E. (1996). The intersubjective perspective. *Psychoanalytic Review*, *83*, 181–194.

Strupp, H. H. (1958). The psychotherapist's contribution to the treatment process. *Behavioral Science*, *3*, 34–67.

Tauber, E. S. (1988). Exploring the therapeutic use of countertransference data. In B. Wolstein (Ed.), *Essential papers on countertransference* (pp. 111–119). New York: New York University Press.

Villard, R. (2013). Skyfire. *Astronomy*, *41*(4), 24–29.

Waska, R. T. (2000). Hate, projective identification, and the psychotherapist's struggle. *Journal of Psychotherapy Practice & Research*, *9*(1), 33–38.

Westen, D., & Gabbard, G. O. (2002). Developments in cognitive neuroscience: II. Implications for theories of transference. *Journal of the American Psychoanalytic Association*, *50*(1), 99–134.

Winnicott, D. W. (1988). Counter-transference. In B. Wolstein (Ed.), *Essential papers on countertransference* (pp. 262–269). New York: New York University Press.

Winnicott, D. W. (1994). Hate in the counter-transference. *Journal of Psychotherapy Practice & Research*, *3*(4), 350–356.

Wolman, B. (Ed.). (1989). *Dictionary of behavioral science* (2nd ed.). San Diego, CA: Academic Press.

Wolstein, B. (1988). Observations of countertransference. In B. Wolstein (Ed.), *Essential papers on countertransference* (pp. 225–261). New York: New York University Press.

Yalom, I. (2002). *The gift of therapy: An open letter to a new generation of therapists and their patients*. New York: Harper Collins.

Zachrisson, A. (2009). Countertransference and changes in the conception of the psychoanalytic relationship. *International Forum of Psychoanalysis*, *18*(3), 177–188.

Zimmermann, J. (2015). *Hermeneutics: A very short introduction*. New York: Oxford University Press.

Zwiebel, R. (1985). The dynamics of the countertransference dream. *International Review of Psychoanalysis*, *12*, 87–99.

Index